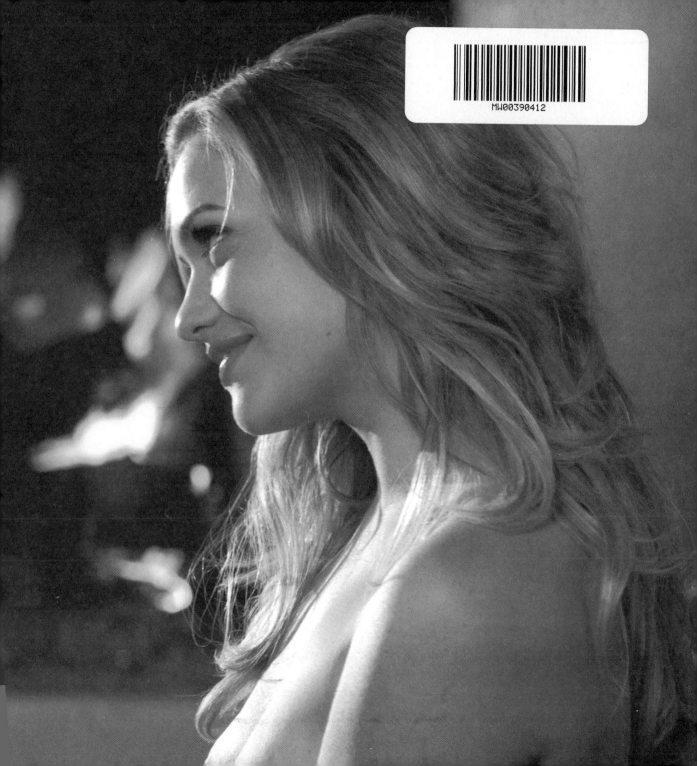

CLASSIC SEX POSITIONS
reinvented

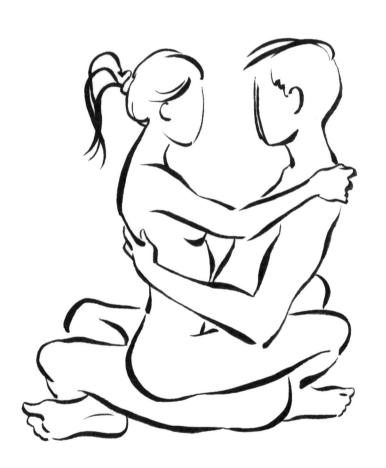

CLASSIC SEX POSITIONS

reinvented

YOUR FAVORITE SEX POSITIONS—100 WILD AND EROTIC WAYS

MOUSHUMI GHOSE, M.A., M.F.T.

FAIR WINDS

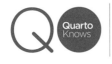

Quarto is the authority on a wide range of topics.

Quarto educates, entertains and enriches the lives of
our readers—enthusiasts and lovers of hands-on living.

www.QuartoKnows.com

© 2016 Quarto Publishing Group USA Inc.
Text © 2016 Moushumi Ghose

First published in the United States of America in 2016 by
Fair Winds Press, an imprint of
Quarto Publishing Group USA Inc.
100 Cummings Center
Suite 406-L
Beverly, Massachusetts 01915-6101
Telephone: (978) 282-9590
Fax: (978) 283-2742
QuartoKnows.com
Visit our blogs at QuartoKnows.com

20 19 18 17 16   1 2 3 4 5

ISBN: 978-1-59233-720-0

Digital edition published in 2016
eISBN: 978-1-63159-165-5

Library of Congress Cataloging-in-Publication Data available

Design: Allison Meierding
Page Layout: Allison Meierding
Photography: Holly Randall
Illustrations (including cover): www.Kathywyatt.com

Printed in China

DEDICATION

This book is dedicated to couples everywhere.
Believe in your strength as a team, while embracing the power
of your individuality, growth, freedom, choice, and change.

CONTENTS

INTRODUCTION

BEING EXCITED AND AROUSED FOR SEX is a wonderful feeling. For the most part, we could say this is half the battle—a requirement, even—but unfortunately, simply wanting sex is not always the be-all and end-all to having great sex. Sometimes, finding creative and fun ways to do it can be a challenge. Sex, like all things, can become monotonous, boring, or lackluster if done often enough in the same way. While not all people get tired of sex, even when they do it a lot, it can be nice to learn a new thing or two. With time our bodies change, and with experience so do our minds. Expanding our sexual repertoire can teach us not only about our partners but also about ourselves.

A book on classic sex positions and their variations is not just for those seeking new variety, adventure, and possibilities. This is also a great guide for beginners who don't know where to start, and for those who are curious about learning about sex and their bodies. But you don't have to be a beginner or seeking excitement. There is something for everyone in these pages.

Some important things to keep in mind as you explore these varieties of sex positions:

- Not every position is going to be great for everyone. Although there is probably a little something for every sexual being within these pages, it is important to remember that everybody is different. Some poses are harder for certain body types. Some poses will stimulate some and won't do anything for others. If something doesn't seem like it is working for you, don't sweat it. Come back to it at a later time, or move on.

- Most sexual poses are easier if you feel comfortable in your environment and are relaxed. It is a little-known fact that when your muscles are relaxed your body is more open and flexible. Feeling safe with your partner helps and, of course, so does being aroused. And the two typically go hand-in-hand.

- Communicate with your partner. This may seem obvious, but it's surprising how much we tend to hold back during sex. Don't hesitate to get the conversation going around sex. Be generous with your words. Ask your partner how it feels, and let him or her know what is working for you and what isn't. Telling your partner ahead of time what you like, dislike, are willing to do, and would like to explore are great ways to break the ice around sex and start building a sexual repertoire together. Communication can also be in the form of body language or moans and groans, which nonverbally suggest that something feels good. Be sure to pay attention to these. Last but not least, dirty talk is also a form of communication, especially when used during sex, and can take each variation to the next level.

- Remember that sex is not only about penetration. Learn to incorporate your hands, fingers, and mouth—not just your genitals. When we go into sex with just the genitals in mind, we inevitably ignore other aspects of feeling and touch. By making sex a full-body experience, we foster mind-body connection. The anus, perineum, testicles, breasts, and nipples (for both men and women) are all highly erogenous zones. Don't ignore these areas!

- Sex does not have to be goal-oriented. The positions in this book focus on man-woman positions, so each variation involves an aspect of intercourse. This does not mean that intercourse must take place for the pose to be successful, nor does it mean that orgasm is a requirement either. Attempting the pose alone can provide a lot of fun and excitement. Remember to enjoy the experience and not focus on the goal of orgasm.

- Speaking of orgasm, considering the fact that most of the poses include an element of penis-vaginal penetration, it is important to note that vaginal orgasms are not the norm for a majority of women. While some women do experience the G-spot orgasm, this is not going to be true for every woman. The G-spot is located inside the vagina, on the anterior wall. More common is the clitoral orgasm.

The clitoris is found outside of the vagina, near the front of her labia and above the urethra. The vagina does have some sensitive spots, such as the G-spot; however, in terms of nerve endings, relatively speaking, the clitoris is much more sensitive.

- Consider adding sex toys to your sexual repertoire. Including toys allows us to think outside of the box and encourages a healthy sexuality that emphasizes growth and learning. When we add toys, we also remind ourselves that sex is about having fun and experimenting with what feels good.

- I can't speak highly enough about lubrication. Whether or not we are naturally lubricated is not necessarily an indication of whether or not we are emotionally aroused. The two are not mutually exclusive. If both partners agree this is something they want, then lube is your best friend. Having a few good types of lube on hand is a good idea. Water-based lubes are best if using condoms. Organic lubes will have the least irritants. Silicone-based lubes will be the slickest, but may not be great when used with silicone toys. Avoid lubes with parabens and glycerin because they can cause irritation. There are a lot of lubes out there, so experiment to find what works for you and your partner.

- Condoms are always a good idea, unless you are in a long-term monogamous relationship, and/or both parties are sharing sexually transmitted disease (STD) sexually transmitted infection (STI) results.

- Another option for safe sex is mutual masturbation. Whether you are touching yourself and/or touching each other, if no fluids are exchanged you are less likely to contract an STI or HIV. Also, mutual masturbation can be a highly erotic experience, connecting two people in a very intimate way. So, definitely don't count this out.

Sex has endless possibilities when you open your mind and let your imagination run wild. So get out there, start exploring, and start growing and learning. Whether you are seeking daring adventures or just trying to learn something new, remember to be safe and have fun!

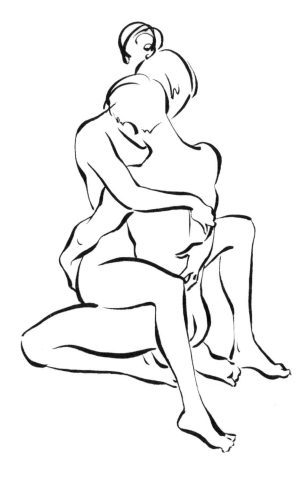

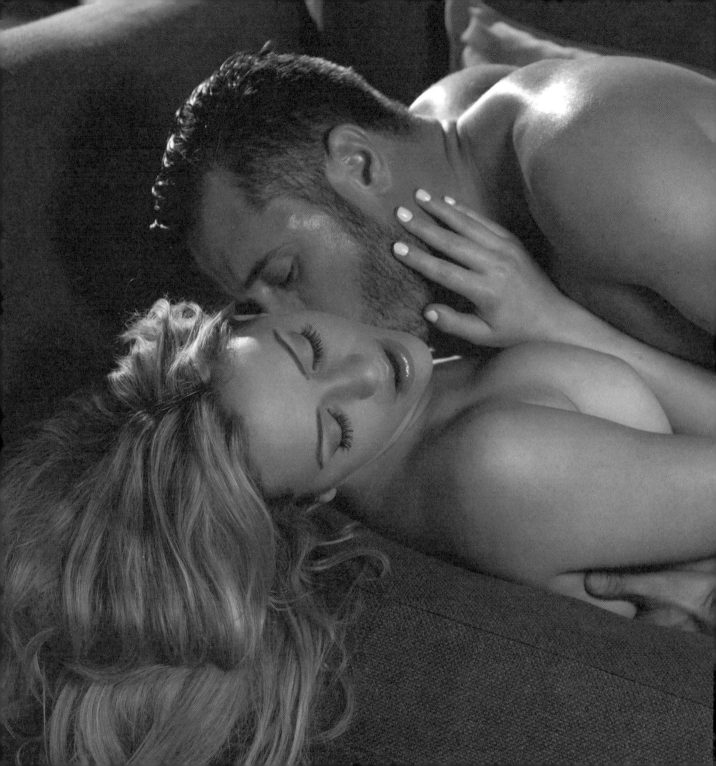

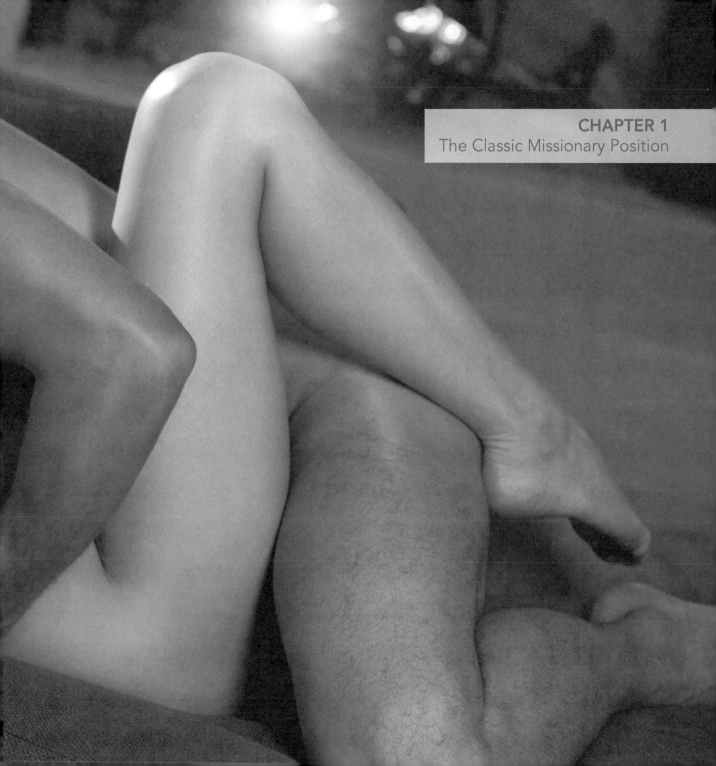

THE CLASSIC MISSIONARY POSITION

I KNOW WHAT YOU'RE THINKING: *The Missionary position? I picked up this book for new ideas—not same-old, same-old!* Bear with me and you will see how truly exciting and profoundly intimate this definitively heterosexual position can be. I know feminists think it relegates the woman to a passive, male-domineering form of sex, but therein lies its beauty. It is perfect when the woman is tired, has had a hard day, or just wants to be ravished by her partner. It is ideal when a man wants to express his powerful masculine side and be more in control. With the man and woman facing each other, this position affords a lot of eye contact, skin-to-skin connection, kissing, and intimacy, which can heighten the senses for a deeply sensual experience during lovemaking. In fact, for a frequently derided "vanilla" position, the Missionary may just be the sexiest and most arousing of them all!

How to Do It

In the traditional Missionary position, the woman lies on her back with her legs spread, either out straight or bent at the knees. The man is also on his knees, facing her, and approaches the woman between her legs. The man can hold himself up with his arms or let his weight rest gently against the woman.

In addition to being a very intimate position, Missionary is thought to promote conception, because the woman being on her back provides a better angle for the sperm to travel toward the uterus and pool in her cervix.

benefits for her

Missionary can be a nice position when she does not have that much energy after a long day, or if she simply would like to take a more passive or submissive role. Taking a submissive role can be especially powerful for a woman who, for example, is typically in control or has a challenging job. This position allows for a sense of complete surrender, which can be a release in and of itself for some women and can connect her to her feminine side, creating a sense of balance.

Although she is underneath him, the woman does have some control and can also increase or decrease the intensity of the thrusting by adjusting her pelvis. For example, moving her pelvis side to side or up and down can increase or decrease the rhythm, creating a variety of experiences for him and her. With her knees bent she can also control the thrusting by digging her feet into the bed, thereby pushing her pelvis up toward him, allowing for deeper penetration, or away from him, for more shallow penetration.

benefits for him

This position is known for allowing easy entrance into the vagina. In this position, the man has most of the control in terms of the degree and intensity of his thrusting and over how deep, shallow, fast, slow, hard, or gentle he goes.

The man can have a sense of power in this position, which can encourage his masculine side and enhance the intensity, not only if dominance is his thing, but also because the woman's trust in him in this position can increase emotional intimacy.

A BIT OF HISTORY

Ancient artifacts from the Greeks, Romans, Indians, and Chinese depict the Missionary position, suggesting that it has been a popular position for a long time. Primates even seem to use this position, further suggesting its primal and instinctive nature.

There is some discrepancy as to how the name *Missionary position* came about. Some believe that the Christian missionaries, when discussing sex, described it as the natural and acceptable position for husband and wife, and would recommend this as the best position for procreation. Others say the first time this term was heard was from Alfred Kinsey in his sex research studies in the early 1950s.

(1.1) MAGIC **BULLET**

In this variation on the Missionary position, termed the Magic Bullet, the man is either on his knees or standing and the woman's legs are straight up in the air. This lets him have a lot more control and access to her vagina, and he will be able to achieve much deeper penetration than in other variations. This position requires a little more strength and flexibility on her part, so it may not be a one that a couple maintains for very long.

what she can do: She can arch her back, reposition her hips, or rest on her elbows or hands to change the angle of the thrusting and increase or decrease the stimulation to her vagina and clitoris.

what he can do: He can hold her legs together while moving in and out, which he can also watch and visually enjoy. He can scissor her legs wide open, then hold her spread legs and act as an anchor for her. He can also better control how deep or shallow he goes.

BONUS!

Why limit yourself to genital-only contact? This position allows him to easily stimulate her clitoris or vagina with his fingers or a vibrator, and she can also stimulate herself or reach down and caress his testicles and the base of his penis. For greater intimacy, he can move her arms above her head and pin them there, then kiss her neck, shoulders, and lips while making smoldering eye contact. What could be hotter?

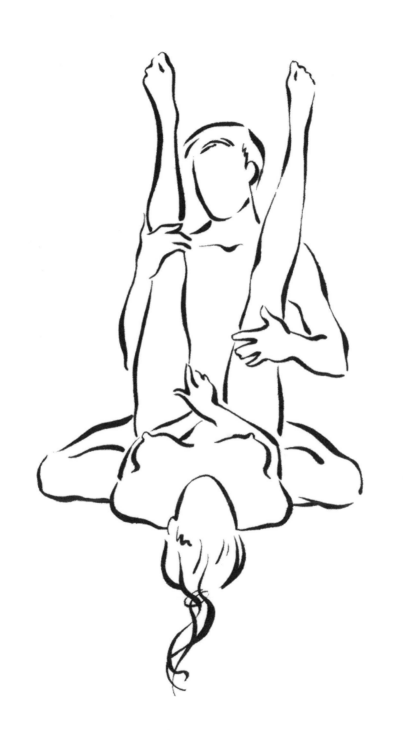

1.2 THE **BUTTERFLY**

In the Butterfly, the woman sits on the edge of the bed or lies back with her legs dangling off the edge. To make penetration easier, she can bend one leg at the knee. He can kneel or stand in front of her. This is an ideal position for that must-have-you-now sex on a countertop, dining table, or desk.

what she can do: If lying down is not an option (such as on a countertop), she can lean back and prop herself up on her elbows for a little more control. Depending on her strength, flexibility, and what feels comfortable, she can either bring her knees back toward her chest for deeper penetration, or she can raise one leg up in a semi-split, with her knee bent. If one foot is actually touching the ground, the split will give her greater control because the grounded leg can provide some stability.

what he can do: This can be a wonderful thrusting position that also stimulates her G-spot. His strength and stamina will determine how long he can stay in this position, as the angle may be difficult to maintain. He can hold on to her hips and pull her onto him for more control as well.

> **BONUS!**
>
> This is an easy position for him to move from standing to crouching, where he has easy access and a full view of her vagina and can vary the stimulation by using his mouth, fingers, or a toy.

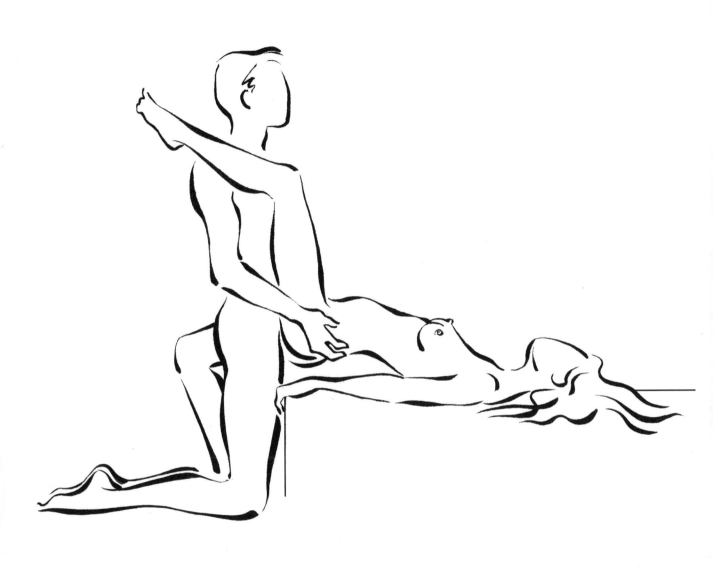

1.3 COITAL **ALIGNMENT TECHNIQUE**

In this variation, the woman brings her legs together between her partner's legs, usually after he is inside her, as initial penetration is difficult in this position. The goal of the Coital Alignment Technique is to encourage the man to slow down and enjoy the ride. The position creates more deliberate movements, which provides the woman more time, direct stimulation of her clitoris, and focus so that she may achieve more intense orgasms during intercourse.

what she can do: The woman can shift her body lower or encourage the man to shift his body forward slightly to make sure there is maximum contact with, and pressure on, her clitoris. A pillow under her hips will lift her pelvis at the correct angle to enjoy the base of his penis thrusting against her clitoris. In fact, this position is often recommended for women who have trouble reaching orgasm during intercourse.

what he can do: In this position, the vagina becomes more constricted and will feel tighter, bringing more sensation to the penis. This is a good position to try after childbirth, when a woman's vagina might feel looser than it previously did. The man can enjoy thrusting in either a horizontal or a vertical motion (a vertical thrusting motion is the cornerstone of the Coital Alignment Technique, but in this position either way may work).

BONUS!

In this position, men learn to slow down and gain more control over ejaculation, which may allow for better timing for the woman so that they both reach orgasm simultaneously.

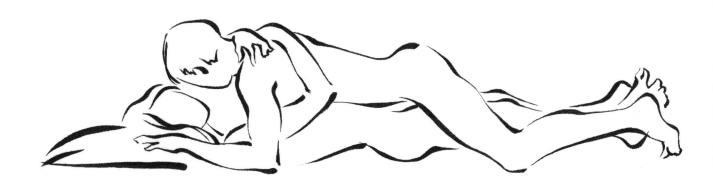

SIDEWAYS MISSIONARY
OR "LOVE-LOCKED"

Once they are in the traditional Missionary position, the couple can roll over
together and enjoy this position on their sides, still facing each other. Or to start
in this position, the man should lie on his side, facing her, with his knees bent and
slightly parted. The woman can lie on her side facing him and gently guide his
penis into her vagina. This position is good for slow and deep contact and greater
intimacy, but it may not be suitable for harder or faster thrusting for prolonged
periods of time.

what she can do: The woman might have to
wiggle and shimmy a little to get the right
angle for penetration. She might wrap her
legs around his torso to gain more traction.
Overall, she has more control in this position because she is not "bed-locked" on
her back, as in the traditional Missionary
position. She can control the rhythm and
intensity of the thrusting and may guide him
by holding his hips.

what he can do: The man can use his fingers
to open the woman's labia and guide his
penis in.

> **BONUS!**
>
> This position allows freer use of
> the hands, so make the most of it.
> Partners can touch and massage
> each other easily, adding to the
> variety of stimulation.

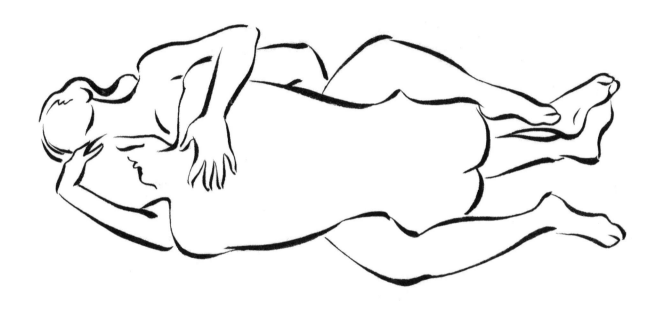

1.5 UPRIGHT **MISSIONARY**

Another great alternative to the classic Missionary position is the Upright Missionary. This intense position often occurs when a couple can't make it to the bedroom and must ravish each other immediately, or when space is tight, such as in a hallway.

In this position, both are standing upright on their feet, face to face. If he is strong enough and/or if she is limber enough, she can wrap her legs around him, while he stabilizes her by wrapping his arms around her waist or holding her up by her hips. From here the thrusting can be very powerful, depending on the strength and stamina of the partners. Upright Missionary maintains all the positives of intimacy, eye contact, and kissing, which build arousal and connection, and the strength required for this position can be a contributing factor to its hotness quotient. By the same token, because there is limited support, this may be a harder position to maintain for longer periods of time.

what she can do: In this position, the support of a wall might be helpful. If he is standing with his back to the wall, she can place her feet against the wall to support herself. Perfect if she is wearing a dress or skirt with no panties, Upright Missionary lends itself to spontaneity and on-the-spot sex.

what he can do: He can lean against a wall to get some leverage for better control and thrusting. Alternatively, he can slide her up against the wall, which can be very sexy and contribute to a feeling of powerful masculinity.

> **BONUS!**
>
> With her pinned up against the wall, it is the perfect time for role-playing a little dominance and surrender.

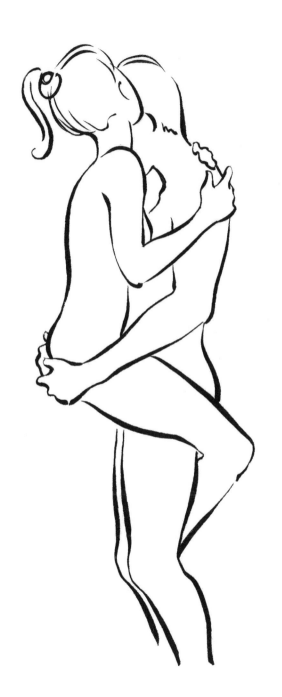

HALF OFF **THE BED**

For a bolder variation of the Missionary position, she can move her body downward so that her lower half falls off the bed while he gets down on his knees in
front of her. This Half Off the Bed variation may occur naturally or accidentally
during lovemaking when they have migrated toward the edge of the bed.

what she can do: She can also hang off the
bed in the opposite direction, with her legs
and butt on the bed and her head and torso
hanging off the bed. This can lead to a rush
of blood to the head and intense orgasms.
If she is far enough down to the ground, she
can lower her arms to the floor in a sort of
handstand position, which may also provide
additional support. However, this position
may put strain on her neck, back, and/or
shoulders, so it is important for her to gently
bring herself back up onto the bed.

what he can do: It is important to be gentle
in this position, especially when bringing her
back up onto the bed. As with all great sex,
this position requires communication, so
make sure she is comfortable before deep
or forceful thrusting.

> **BONUS!**
>
> This position makes her easily
> accessible for oral sex. He can
> slide down to pleasure her with his
> mouth and hands.

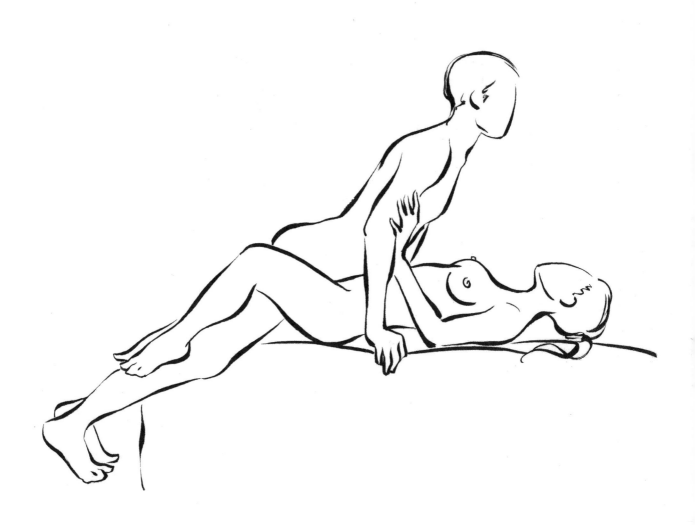

STANDING **MISSIONARY**

In this position, the man is standing up while the woman is still on her back. He is either kneeling on the bed or standing between her legs as she lies with her torso on the bed and her legs over the edge. Her legs are bent for better leverage, and she can rest her feet on his chest or shoulders or on the bed.

what she can do: Because his body is not hovering directly above hers, she can be a little more flexible with her moves. She can also lean up on her elbows to get a better view of the action. For more direct contact with her G-spot, he can place a pillow under her lower back to raise her pelvis toward him. In a slight variation, she can wrap her legs around his body to bring him closer toward her, which will help her control the thrusting and the depth of penetration. She can also caress his arms, chest, and shoulders (if she can reach) and play with his nipples.

what he can do: In this position, the man has an excellent view of all that's happening, including watching his penis moving in and out of her vagina. He also has perfect access to caress her breasts or stimulate her clitoris. He can kiss and massage her feet and legs as well.

> **BONUS!**
>
> While he watches from his standing vantage point, she can stimulate herself with her hands or a vibrator.

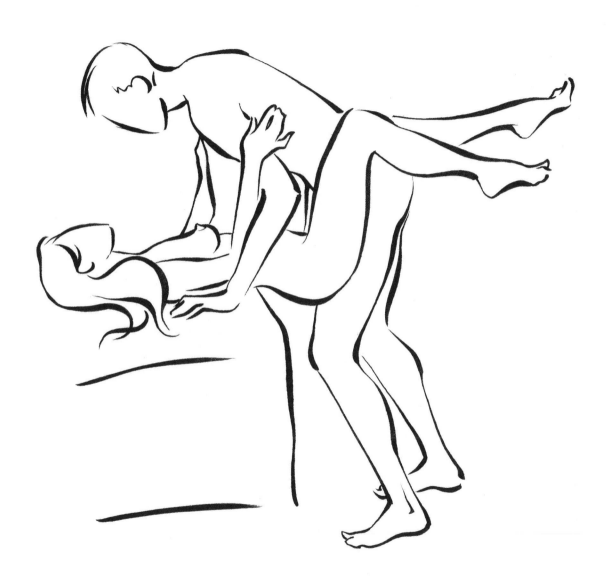

(1.8) THE SEASHELL

In this variation, she is on her back with her legs up over her head. She can cross them at the ankles if it feels more comfortable, but that may require a bit more flexibility. He can enter her from the same angle as in the Missionary position, with his knees still on the bed, and help keep her legs pushed back by gently shifting his weight onto her.

what she can do: Placing a pillow under her lower back will elevate her pelvis for more direct contact with her clitoris and deeper penetration.

what he can do: He can move up higher so that his pelvic bone and the shaft of his penis rub against her clitoris, or he can lower himself to an angle that will stimulate her G-spot with the head of his penis. He can also rock back and forth in a deliberately slow and gentle movement to build tension for a more powerful orgasm.

> **BONUS!**
>
> If she is comfortable with a bit of anal this is a good position for him to stimulate her anus with his finger. Remember, though, that it is very important to go slow, and by slow this could mean days, weeks, or months before she is ready for anal penetration, if ever. It is always best to start with one finger. And of course, lube is absolutely essential, as the anus has no natural lubrication of its own.

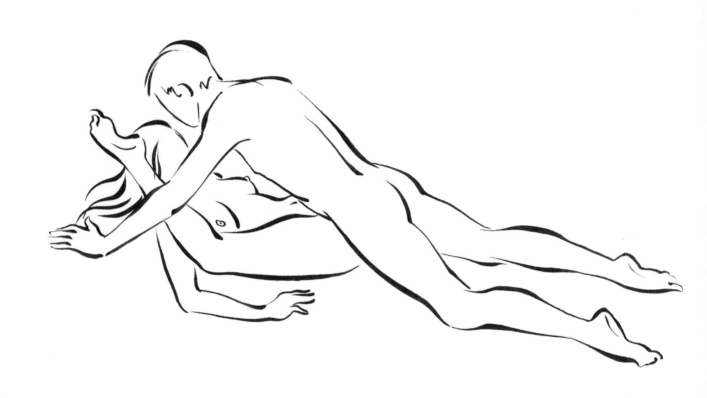

1.9 THE **MAN** TRAP

Another way to vary the Missionary position is for the woman to wrap her legs around his body or around his calves, essentially trapping him against her.

what she can do: She can try squeezing her legs together, allowing for more direct stimulation to her clitoris, while also providing a tighter sensation for him. She may wrap her arms around him to pull his body close, or grab his hips to control the speed of his thrusting and the angle of penetration.

what he can do: Even though he is on top, her strong legs wrapped around his torso give her more control and changes the power dynamic. He can respond by taking a more submissive role and following her lead.

BONUS!

Get playful or kinky by using scarves, ties, or handcuffs to bind her hands above her head for a role-playing scenario or for a sense of submission and surrender. She can try spanking him to increase momentum or pleasure.

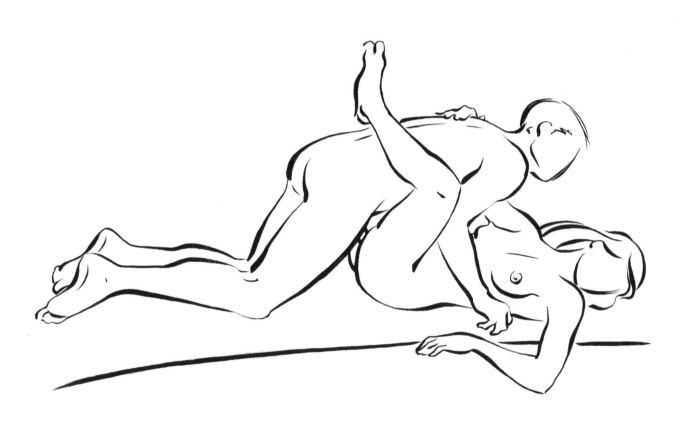

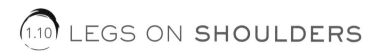

1.10 LEGS ON **SHOULDERS**

For this variation, he can either kneel down or sit upright on his ankles, or he can be in a standing position. While she is lying on her back, he enters her and guides her legs up onto both of his shoulders. He can then support her hips for powerful thrusting.

what she can do: She can move her legs off of his shoulders and in front of his face and then squeeze her legs closed, which will more directly stimulate her clitoris and tighten her vagina around his penis. Or she can spread her legs apart as they rest on his shoulders for a different angle and depth of penetration.

what he can do: This position may be more tiring for her because her legs are raised, but he can continue to support her legs with his hands or let her rest them on his shoulders. He can shift her legs from one shoulder to the other, so that his penis massages the sides of her vagina.

> **BONUS!**
>
> He has a great view for watching himself going in and out of her. Place a standing mirror near the bed so she can enjoy the show, too.

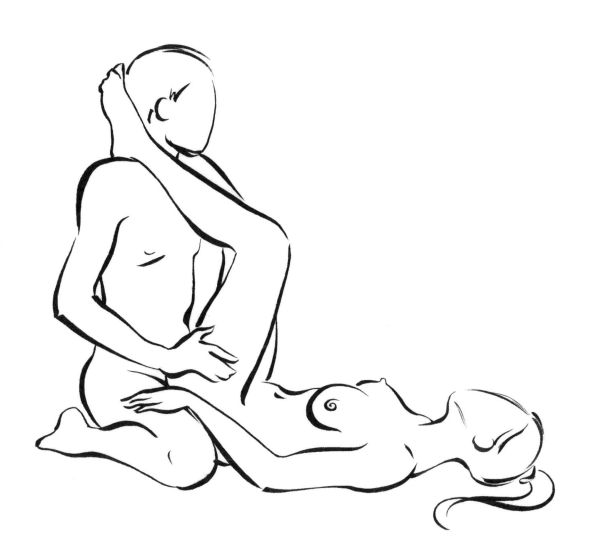

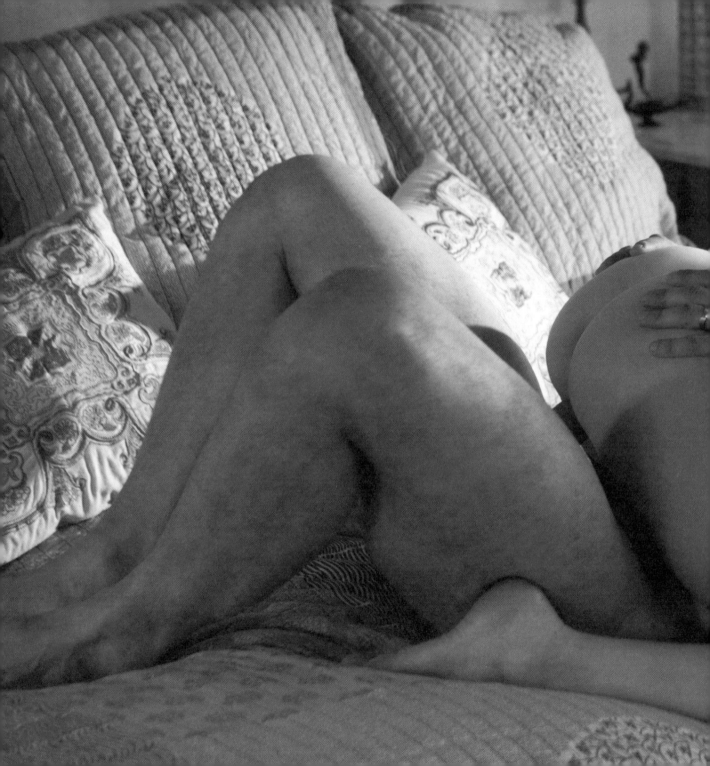

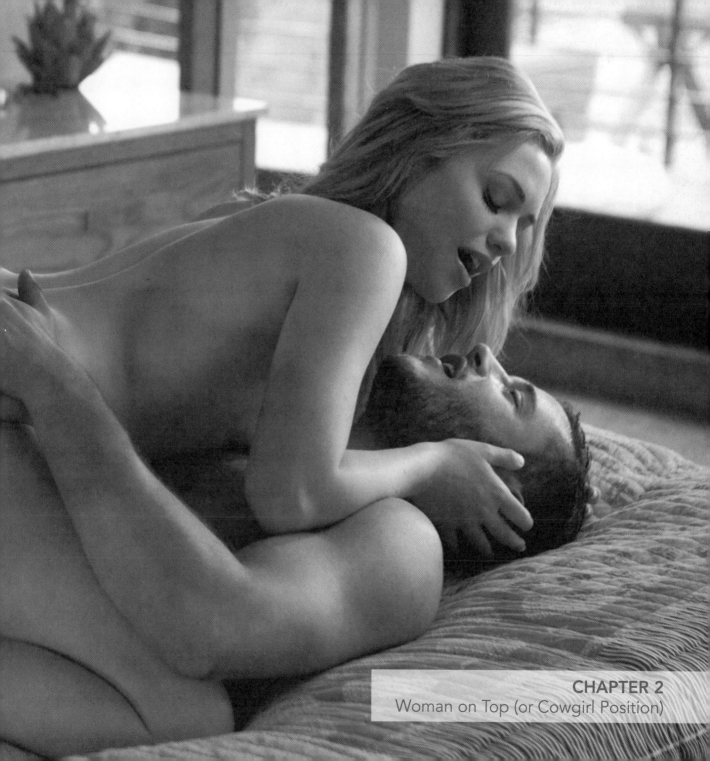

CHAPTER 2
Woman on Top (or Cowgirl Position)

WOMAN ON TOP (OR COWGIRL POSITION)

WOMAN ON TOP OR COWGIRL are a group of sex positions in which the man lies on his back or is sitting. As the name suggests, the woman is on top, straddling him. This position offers a lot of variety and the woman has more control over rhythm, vigor, and depth of penetration. These positions also emphasize a woman's pleasure, as they suggest that she knows how to satisfy herself and is happy to take the reins, "riding" her partner as a cowgirl rides a bucking horse or bull.

How to Do It

He lies on his back, sits up on the edge of the bed, or leans back against a wall or the headboard of the bed. She rises up on her knees and either flings a leg across his hips or straddles him at his feet and inches up his body with one knee on each side. This is a great seductress move that builds anticipation. She then guides his penis into her and initiates the movement. From this position she can easily slide down between his legs and give him some oral pleasure or move her hips up over his face to enjoy some cunnilingus.

benefits for her

Although it may be tempting to mimic the traditional male-dominant position and head right into fast thrusting, she can opt to start slowly, moving in deliberate, circular motions until she gets a comfortable rhythm going. She can vary the stimulation with up-and-down and forward-and-backward movements, alternating between shallow and deep thrusts. She can angle herself so that his penis perfectly hits her G-spot, penetrates her vagina more deeply, or rubs against her clitoris. This is also a great time to tease him by raising her hips and letting his penis slide out until he is begging for deeper contact.

benefits for him

The man can appreciate lying back and letting her take control. It's a great position for her to show him what she likes and for him to follow her lead. He can stimulate her clitoris as she rides him and also fondle and kiss her breasts. For greater stability, he can hold her at the waist and move her up and down to his liking, switching up the power dynamic.

A GOOD POSITION DURING PREGNANCY

This is a great position for pregnant women who can't have a man lying on top of them or whose skin or breasts are especially sensitive to touch. No matter how big her belly gets, she can always find a way to straddle him, and because she is on top she can direct his hands where she wants them—or hold his hands above his head for a show of dominance that also ensures he won't touch her swollen, tender breasts.

2.1 REVERSE **MISSIONARY**

From the kneeling position of Cowgirl, she leans forward into the position known as Reverse Missionary. This is essentially a more intimate position than Cowgirl, because both partners are face to face and can embrace, caress, and kiss each other. This position creates a natural angle for the penis to enter directly into the vagina. Both partners can thrust, and it's a little less tiring for the woman than sitting straight up.

what she can do: From the Cowgirl position, the woman simply leans forward until she is lying on her partner's chest. Stretching out her legs behind her will put more pressure on her clitoris. She can grind her clitoris against him and maneuver herself so that his penis is angled toward her G-spot.

what he can do: He can still be in charge from this position, even though he is underneath. He can grab hold of her hips or her butt to get better control of the thrusting and to help guide her motions. He might also do this to give her a break, or when he wants to speed things up for his pleasure or orgasm.

> **BONUS!**
>
> If the woman stretches her legs out behind her, the man can separate his legs, so that she can put her legs between his. By pressing her thighs together in this position she can increase the tightness on his penis. It is also a nice change from always having her legs on the outside of his.

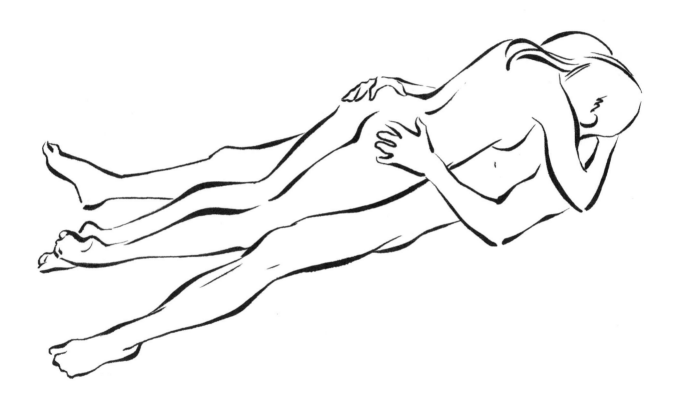

(2.2) LAP **DANCE**

This variation is both fun and sexy but has the potential to be intimate as well. The face-to-face nature of this position makes it ideal for caressing, eye contact, and kissing. She takes the lead by sitting him down on a chair, a couch, or the edge of the bed. As she faces him, she climbs onto his lap. If the couple is already in the woman-on-top position (Cowgirl or Reverse Missionary), he can just sit upright, so that she is essentially sitting in his lap.

what she can do: Her weight is on his thighs, and she may try placing her legs on his shoulders, if she is flexible. She may also place her hands on his thighs or the back of the chair to control the thrusting. She can hold on to his shoulders and lean back, move her hips closer to his torso and wrap her arms around his neck for a more intimate embrace, or bounce up and down on him. She can also move down onto her knees between his legs and put her lips around his penis, looking up into his eyes as she takes it in her mouth.

what he can do: He can pull her hips back and forth to assist with or control the speed of thrusting. Leaning back will change the angle of penetration.

> **BONUS!**
>
> If she wants to keep her underwear on, and he keeps his clothes on, this position is great for a bit of teasing with a little more coverage, such as if she visits him in his office for a little afternoon delight. Alternatively, she can unleash her inner stripper and get creative with props, sexy lingerie, and even dance moves.

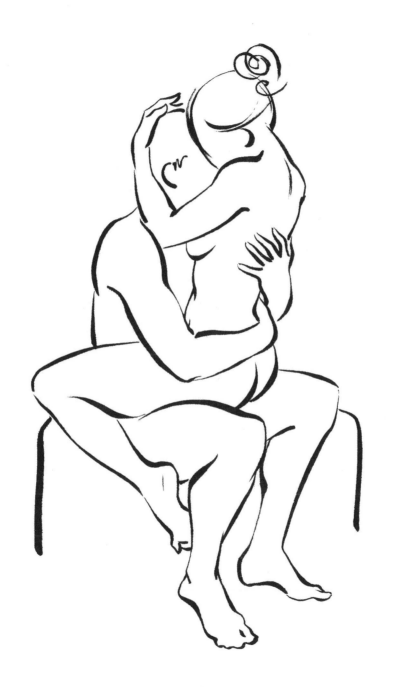

2.3 REVERSE **LAP DANCE**

In this position, both the man and the woman are sitting upright, preferably in a chair. To get into the position, he sits down first with his legs slightly spread, then she backs up into him and sits down on his lap, facing away from him.

what she can do: This position retains all the excellent qualities of woman-on-top positions. She is still in control and can move her hips side to side or up and down. Arching her back will stimulate her G-spot, and squeezing her thighs together will provide a tighter feel. By leaning forward or backward, she can change the angle of penetration.

what he can do: He gets to sit back, let her take the reins, and enjoy the view. His hands are free, so he can play with her breasts, rub her clitoris, or hold on to her hips to help participate in the movements and thrusting. He can also nibble on her neck, shoulders, and ears.

> **BONUS!**
>
> She can engage her inner exotic dancer and try more sensual moves on him. How about giving him a striptease as a precursor? Role-playing can be a fun option, too: Perhaps he is a paying customer, or a stranger whom she never sees and doesn't know.

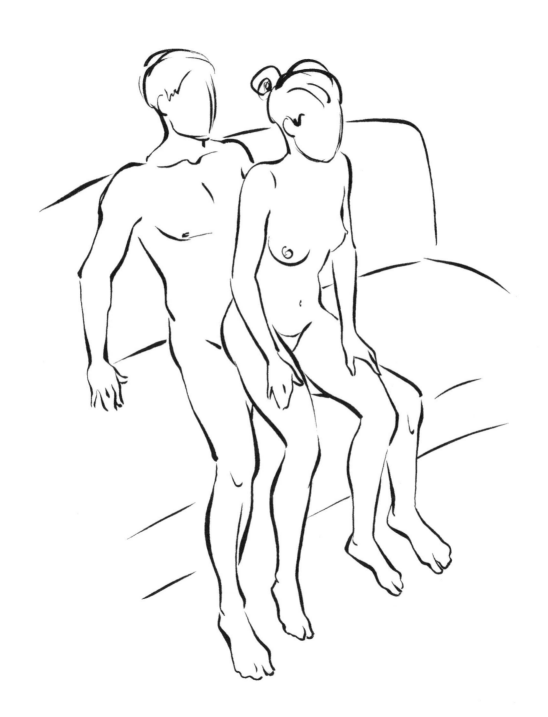

2.4 THE **DOUBLE DECKER**

If the man is on the bed for the Reverse Lap Dance, it is easy to transition to the Double Decker, but this variation is also an easy one to get into from any woman-on-top position. He lies face up on his back and she first sits down on top of him, facing away from him, toward his feet. She leans back until she's propped up on her elbows, her back on his chest, with her arms supporting her body weight.

what she can do: If she keeps her knees bent and places her feet up on his knees, it makes access to her vagina and penetration a little easier because she has a bit more leverage and control. To increase her pleasure, she can prop up on one arm and use the other hand to stimulate her nipples or clitoris with her fingers or a vibrator.

what he can do: The man can hold her at the waist to help stabilize his thrusting. Although she is on top, this position allows him to control the rhythm. To add some sensuality, he can kiss her neck, ears, and shoulders while thrusting. From this vantage point, he can see her body as it reacts to his thrusting for a completely different visual experience. His hands are free to stimulate her breasts and clitoris and run his hands up and down her body.

> **BONUS!**
>
> The Double Decker is a good transition position because it's easy for the man to roll the woman over and into a new position, such as onto her stomach, where he can enter her from behind or engage in some anal play.

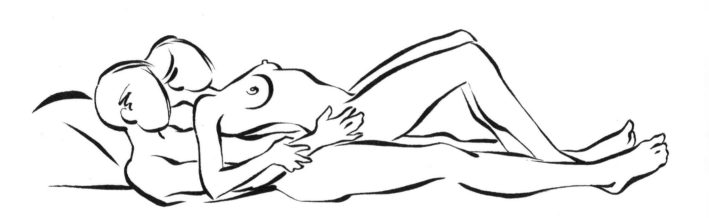

2.5 THE **FROG**

This position is also known as the *squat* and is a slight variation from the Lap Dance. The man should be on a bed or a wide chair or couch for this position to work. Instead of kneeling, the woman straddles him, plants her feet on the bed, and literally squats down onto his penis. She may hold her body straight up or lean forward. This can feel great for both partners. The angle of her pelvis being somewhat upright provides leverage and makes it easier for his penis to go straight up into her vagina.

what she can do: Depending on her strength, and with his help in holding her up and in place, she can use a vibrator to massage her clitoris, while he controls the thrusting. However, this position can get tiring if the thrusting becomes faster and harder, which can also feel awkward for her if she is trying to keep her balance. This position may not be ideal for longer periods of time.

what he can do: The man can help out by holding the woman's butt up with his hands or thighs, or he can hold her up by bracing her hips. From here he can move her up and down onto his penis and control the motion and speed of thrusting.

> **BONUS!**
>
> He has a great view and can see his erect penis going in and out of her vagina, which provides visual stimulation and extended arousal. If she can maintain this position for a greater length of time, it can also lead to powerful orgasms.

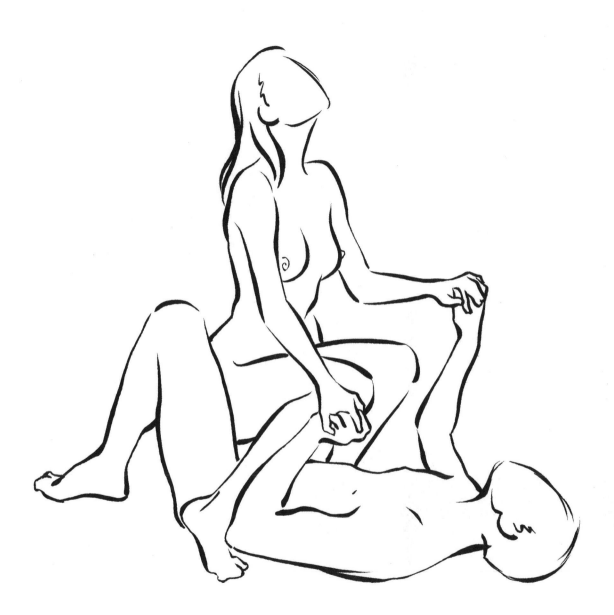

2.6 THE SHIP

With the man lying on his back, the woman sits to one side of him, then raises her hips above him and lowers herself down onto his penis. Both legs remain on one side of his torso, with her at a 90-degree angle to his body.

what she can do: She has immense control in this position. She can sit cross-legged, have her legs spread or bent, or squat above him.

what he can do: Because she is doing much of the work in this position, he can take a breather but still caress her back, neck, and nipples.

BONUS!

His hands have equal access to her clitoris and anus, and caressing them simultaneously can lead to an explosive orgasm for her.

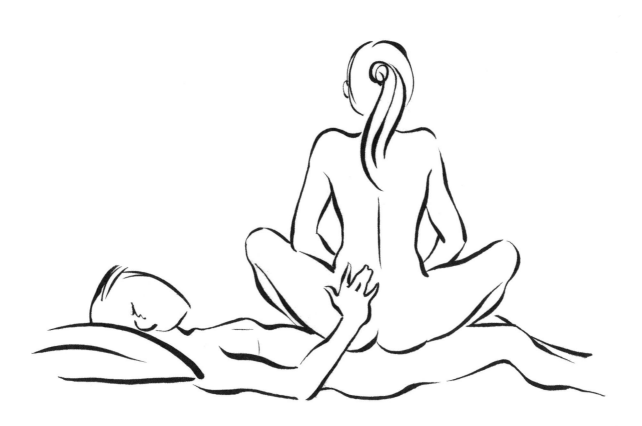

(2.7) REVERSE ISIS

From the Ship position, where he is lying on his back, she turns herself another 90 degrees to face his feet and straddles his hips, lowering herself onto his penis. He may have straight legs or knees bent, depending on which is more comfortable or better suited for penetration.

what she can do: She can control the thrusting by using her leg and thigh muscles to move herself up and down. She can use her hands for support by placing them in front on his legs or on the bed, or reach back and put her hands on his thighs. She can look back over her shoulder and make eye contact as well.

what he can do: Besides just sitting back and enjoying the ride, he can play with her breasts, stimulate her clitoris, or simply hold her hips and guide her motions to give her a rest. He can also raise himself up onto his elbows for more support and to get a better view.

> **BONUS!**
>
> This is a great position for her to experiment with a variety of movements, such as gyrating her hips back and forth or moving round and round in circles. By moving her upper body forward she can give him an excellent visual of her backside, and if she arches her back her G-spot may get stimulated.

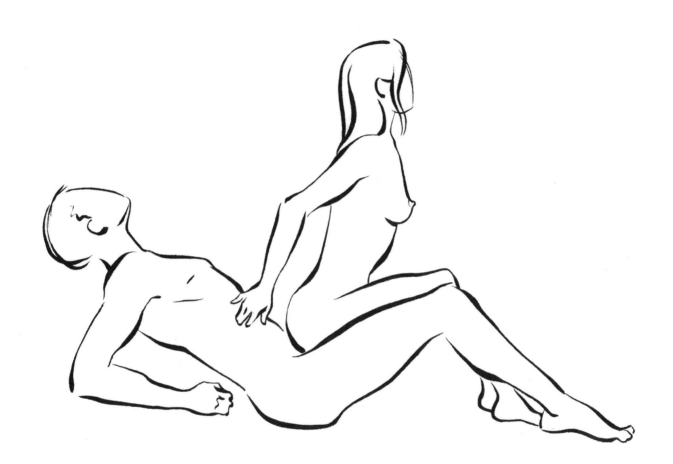

REVERSE **COWGIRL**

The popular Cowgirl position can also be reversed for a variation known as Reverse Cowgirl. The main difference from Reverse Cowgirl and Reverse Isis is that in Reverse Cowgirl, her legs are bent and she is sitting on her knees.

what she can do: Her strength comes from her thighs and knees in this position. She can move forward and put her weight onto her hands to aid with the thrusting. This will also give him a nice view of her backside. It is important to pay attention to the curvature of his penis. For example, if his penis naturally curves upward and toward him, she might lean back toward his chest. This may have the effect of hitting her G-spot.

what he can do: He can control the action by holding her hips to guide her up and down. He may also prop his head up with pillows or prop himself up on his elbows, changing the angle of penetration.

> ### BONUS!
>
> Her being on top and in control, as with all woman-on-top positions, can give him an added sense of submission or surrender, and her one of power and dominance. If this is something that both partners enjoy exploring, they can play it up with dirty talk, role-playing, or props.

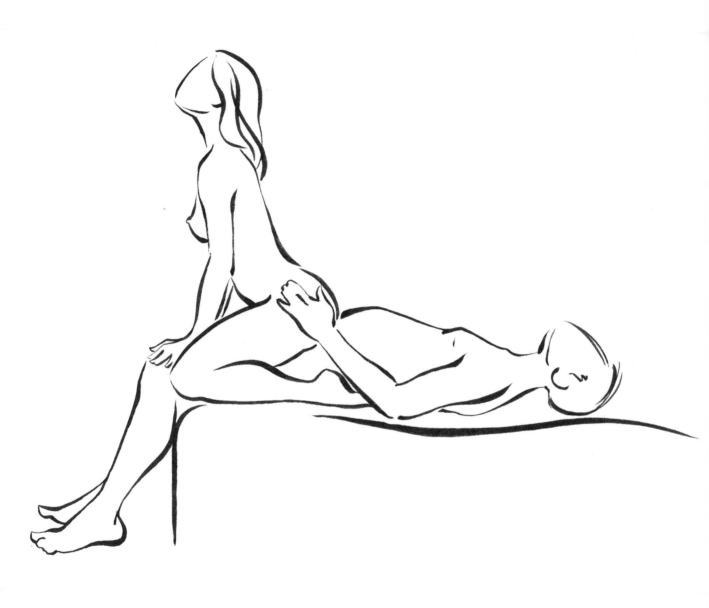

REVERSE FROG
OR REVERSE SQUAT

If she is already in a Reverse Cowgirl, she just brings her legs out from under her and places her feet on the bed, still facing away from him. She can also get into this position from standing, simply by straddling him and coming down into a squat. He can be sitting upright with his legs hanging off the bed, or he can be lying down. His head can be propped up with pillows or he can use his elbows and arms to bring his body closer to hers.

what she can do: She has complete power to experiment and to take the lead. She also controls the rhythm, speed, and motion of penetration. For more balance and control, she can place her hands in front of her and arch her back to change the angle of penetration.

what he can do: He can hold on to her hips to guide the thrusting to his liking. In this position, he gets excellent visuals of his penis going in and out of her as she lifts her hips and lowers them.

BONUS!

The curvature of his penis plays a role in this position, so while it is important to make sure this is a comfortable angle for him, it can also be an excellent way to discover and stimulate erogenous zones within the vagina.

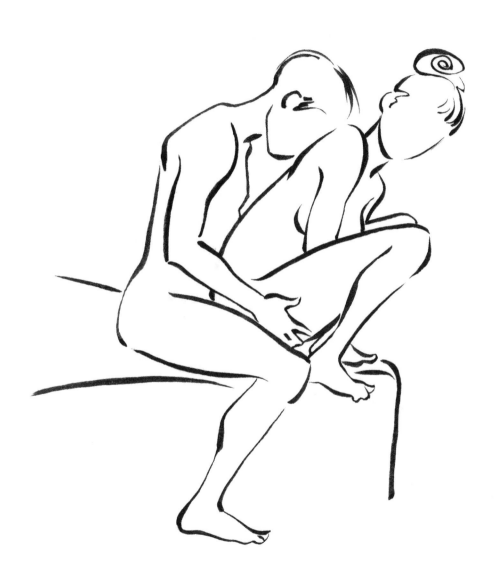

(2.10) THE STALLION

In this position, he lies flat on his back with his knees bent and legs spread apart. He can prop himself up on his elbows if he wants. Facing away from him, she gets on top of him and lowers herself down, keeping her knees bent. The key to riding the Stallion is leaning forward on his legs, which support her. From here he can thrust his hips up and down.

what she can do: Leaning forward will provide balance and control to maintain the position. She can use her arms to push herself up and down as well. This angle is great for hitting the G-spot, while her clitoris rubs against his body, which stimulates two highly sensitive areas simultaneously. She can move her hips around or side to side to hit different angles.

what he can do: In this position, he has an excellent view of her backside and the motion of going in and out of her. He can hold her hips to control the speed of the thrusting. He is also in the perfect position for some anal play, which will hit three of her erogenous zones at once.

BONUS!

This position is a shared effort. Although she is on top, he has a little more control than other woman-on-top positions. Communication is key here, because the partners are facing away from each other and can't maintain eye contact or watch each other's faces for clues. Sharing responsibility for mutual pleasure can strengthen the bond between them.

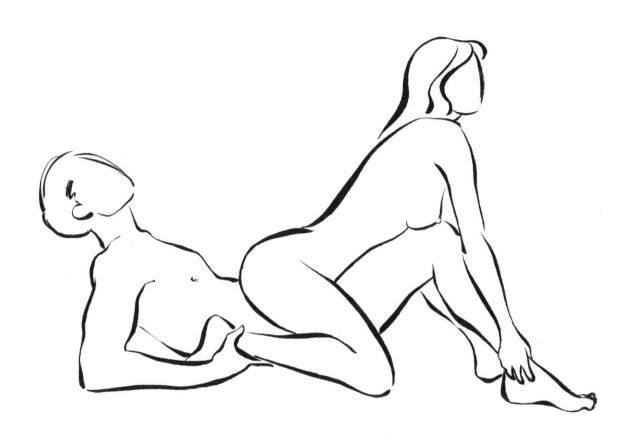

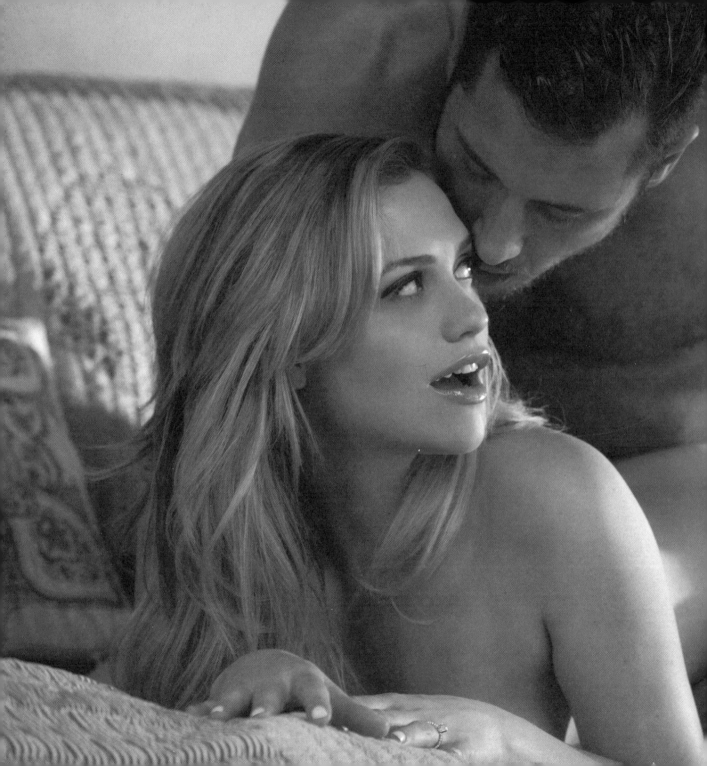

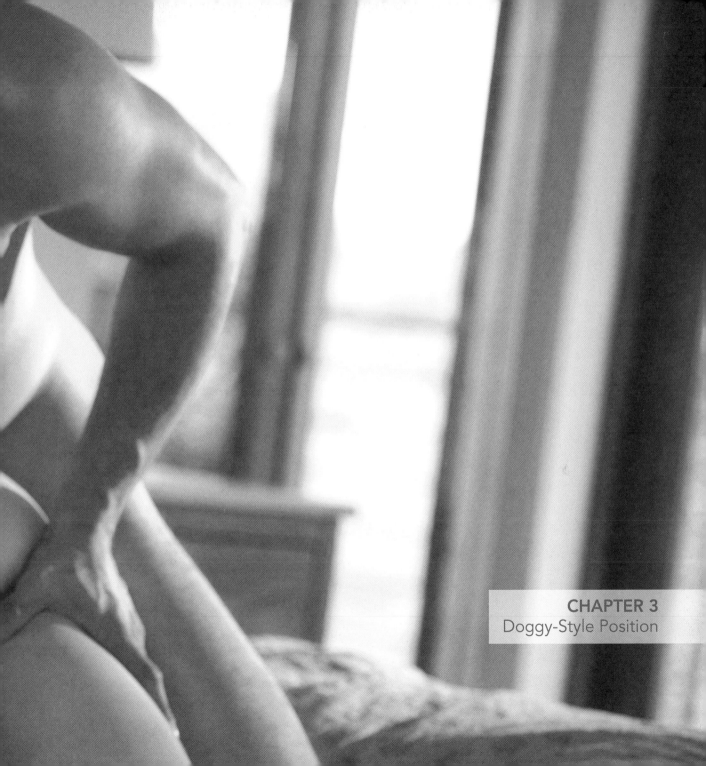

CHAPTER 3
Doggy-Style Position

DOGGY-STYLE POSITION

DOGGY STYLE, ALSO REFERRED TO AS REAR ENTRY, is a group of sex positions where the woman is on her hands and knees and the man enters her vagina from behind her. In this position, he is seen as taking on the more dominant role, whereas the woman is often seen as the passive recipient. The variations of Doggy Style are often based on shifting her hips, butt, and arms for varied angles and depth of penetration.

Men often enjoy this position because he can see his penis moving in and out of her, and from this angle his penis may look quite large, a huge ego boost to his sense of virility. Some who are having casual sex may prefer the more distant nature of this position, which precludes eye contact and intimate kissing. Because of the lack of clitoral stimulation, some women cite this as their least favorite and even a boring position. However, with the right position and some encouragement from a vibrator, a hand, or a well-placed pillow, this can be a highly arousing and satisfying position for both partners. And doing it in front of the mirror can be a pretty fine work-around for the lack of eye contact.

How to Do It

She may be on all fours on the bed, and he can stand behind her on the floor or kneel behind her on the bed. Her back is flat like a tabletop with her ass scooted back toward his penis. He can grab hold of her hips and control the thrusting. If her knees are getting tired, she can kneel on a pillow.

benefits for her

Because of the deep penetration possible in this position, it may be better for G-spot stimulation. If she can balance on one arm she can stimulate her clitoris, or she can ask him to reach around and stimulate it for her, or she can use a vibrator or grind against a pillow. Men like the easy access of this position, so to titillate him even further, she can wear a dress without panties and simply lift it up in the back to show him what she has in mind.

benefits for him

This position affords a great view of the vagina from a different angle and can feel slightly animalistic, which can heighten arousal. He can pull her hips toward him as he thrusts, emphasizing feelings of power and dominance.

THE EVOLUTION OF DOGGY STYLE

The origin of the term *doggy style* points to the idea that the position is seen in the animal kingdom. The Latin name for this position, *coitus more ferarum*, translates to "sexual intercourse in the manner of wild beasts" and in the Kama Sutra, an ancient Indian text on sexual positions, it is known as the *cow position*. In most evolutionary works it is thought to be common among primates. Due to the lack of eye contact in the Doggy-Style position, some believe that humans biologically evolved out of this sex position in search of something that promoted intimacy and thus fostered stable, long-term relationships.

DOGGY **ANGLE**

Doggy Angle is a great position to transition to when she is on all fours. It does not require as much strength or flexibility as the classic position, and she gets more clitoral stimulation in this one. In the Doggy Angle position, the woman is face down on the bed. She may be propped up on her forearms, with her hands framing her head and neck for support. If this is the case, she should turn her head to either the right side or the left so as not to put strain on her neck. A pillow may be used under her belly for support. She then raises her butt up in the air, so that he can easily enter her. He will have his legs close together inside hers.

what she can do: When in this position, it may seem as though the man is doing most of the work, but she can also thrust back against him to control the depth of penetration and for more vigorous sex. Also, she's in an easy position to stimulate her clitoris. By leaning forward or backward, she can raise or lower her hips, which will create different angles of entry. Changing the height of her butt can also vary the angle at which he enters her.

what he can do: He can also change the angle of penetration by leaning either backward or forward. He can place his hands on her back while thrusting, or he can grab her hips so that he can thrust with more force. He is also in a great position to provide some manual stimulation with his hands, by reaching over to touch her clitoris.

BONUS!

With her lovely ass raised in the air, this is a good time to engage in some light spanking. Some people enjoy a bit of erotic pain during lovemaking because it ups the sexual charge. Some couples enjoy S&M games to switch up their routines or act out fantasies. Just make sure she's into it first. Sadomasochism, better known as S&M (sadism and masochism) is a form of sexual play involving pain, punishment, and/or psychological control. While this may be a single sexual act, this is also often used more broadly as a lifestyle involving psychological power play and dynamics such as Master & Servant. These should be carried out between consenting adults only.

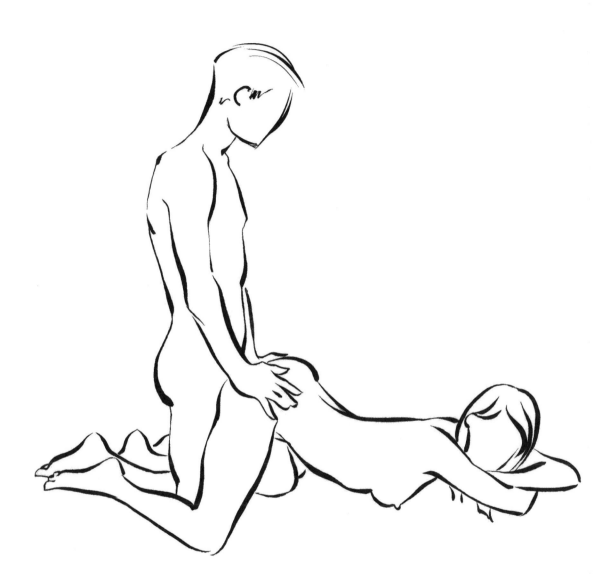

3.2 FLYING **DOGGY**

In this position, similar to the classic Doggy Style, she is either on all fours or is standing; he is standing behind her or on his knees. The cornerstone of this position is that he holds her wrists behind her back, as if cuffed together.

what she can do: She can bend over, pushing her pelvis back against him and allowing for easier and deeper penetration. Having her hands restrained behind her back allows her to experience complete submission, which can be very erotic. This position allows for really deep penetration, which can be uncomfortable for some women. If this is the case, she can try bringing her legs closer together, which will result in shallower penetration. On the other hand, if she loves deep penetration, spreading her legs apart will allow him to go deeper.

what he can do: Holding her hands back may play into his desire to control and dominate during sex. He can also shift his weight and the angle at which she is leaning forward to vary the stimulation.

> **BONUS!**
>
> Of course, this position lends itself to erotic role-play. Some women enjoy the fantasy of being overtaken by someone stronger, thus releasing them of "responsibility" for sex. He can tie her hands together with a scarf or bathrobe belt to increase the power play.

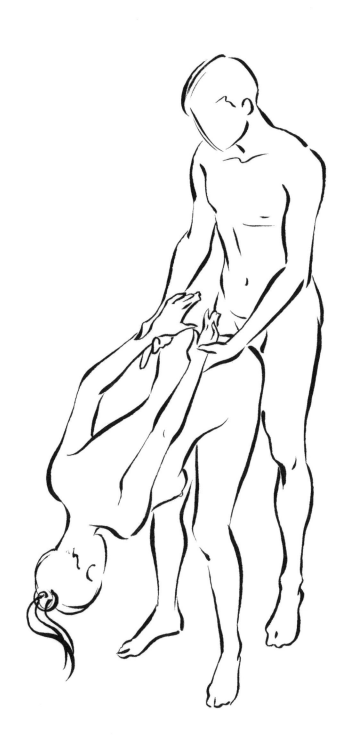

FROGGY **STYLE**

This variation is similar to Doggy Style; however, instead of crouching on all fours and being on her knees, she squats on her feet like a frog. She is supporting her weight with her leg muscles, requiring some degree of stamina and strength on her part. The man kneels behind her and for rear entry. It may look and feel like she is ready to jump!

what she can do: She may find this position gets tiring very quickly, so she can support herself with her hands. She can push her butt up toward him or lower it to the ground to see which angle suits her best. As with many of the Doggy variations, direct eye contact will require that she look back over her shoulder at him.

what he can do: This position may or may not be good for him depending on his height. If it is a good height for him, he can play around with this variation to find the right angle. He can hold on to her hips and slide in and out of her. He can also press his torso forward; if his hands are free, he can caress her back, breasts, and clitoris.

> **BONUS!**
>
> Mixing it up a little can add fun to any position. Try putting a blindfold on her, or both can use a blindfold. This heightens the senses and focuses attention inward.

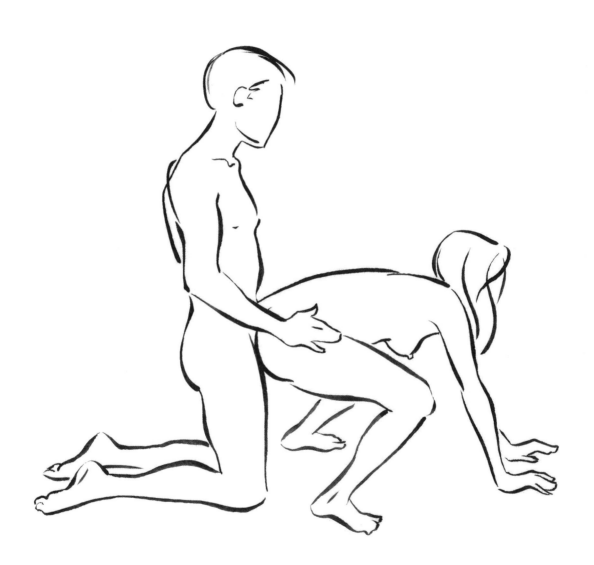

(3.4) THE **PLOW**

In this slightly more edgy version of Doggy Style she lies with her head and chest on the bed and her legs and hips extending off the bed. He is in between her legs and can grab hold of her hips to bring her ass closer to him. In this position she will be supporting her body weight up on her elbows.

what she can do: She can play up this submissive role by looking back at him over her shoulder and complimenting him on his moves. Talking dirty is another way to enhance this kind of play. Using words that imply subservience or authority can heighten the power play and intensify the position.

what he can do: This position provides great visuals and the feeling of being in control. Because she is only partially on the bed, he is holding her up and is her main support. This requires a lot of trust on her part, so he should make sure that she is comfortable and not in danger of falling. If there is room, he can take a step or two back, pulling her with him slightly, but she must hold on tight so that she doesn't hit her head if he goes too far.

> **BONUS!**
>
> Sex does not have to be confined to just the bed. This position can be done from the couch or the kitchen countertop. Just make sure she has enough room for her head and upper torso, as she is elongated in this position.

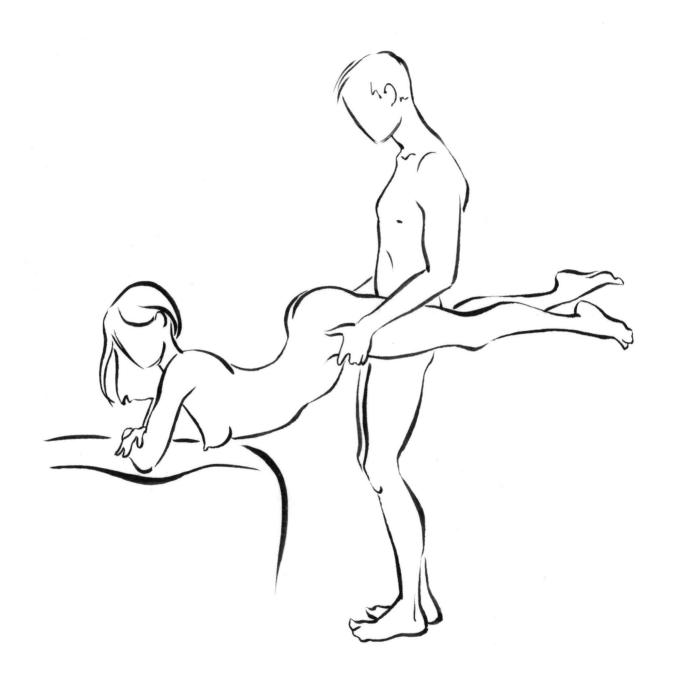

(3.5) THE **MAGIC MOUNTAIN**

Using props can be another way to vary the Doggy-Style position. In this position the man and woman essentially construct a "mountain" out of a pile of firm pillows. The woman kneels in front of the pillows and leans over them. The man kneels behind her, while his legs are outside of hers. He then leans down over her and enters her from behind.

what she can do: This position retains all the thrills of original Doggy Style while the pillows provide a soft landing for her. Adjusting her body can slightly alter the angle of penetration. She can move forward to elevate her body a little higher, so that he is almost lying on top of her, or she can move backward until she is sitting in his lap. She may also try turning her head to kiss him on the lips.

what he can do: With all that padding underneath her, he may just be able to go full force with his thrusting. Because he drapes himself over her, there is a whole lot more skin-to-skin contact in this position, making it a sensual intimacy builder. From this position he can easily kiss her neck, shoulders, and ears.

> **BONUS!**
>
> If both partners enjoy the comfort and ease that a mountain of pillows provides, they might consider purchasing sex pillows and ramps made exactly for this purpose. They come in a range of colors and styles, with zip-off covers for easy washing.

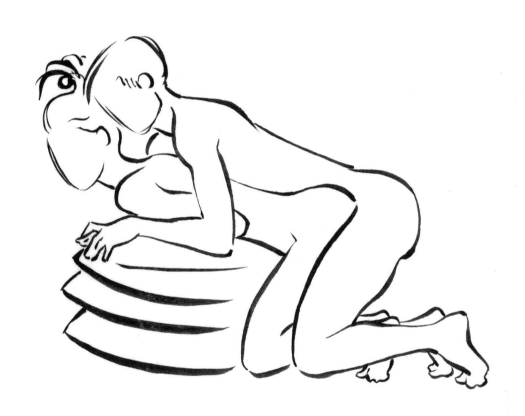

(3.6) THE **FAN**

Legs getting tired? Stretching them out and getting up off the floor while also using another prop provides a standing variation of Doggy Style. The woman stands in front of a chair, stool, couch, or desk with her back to her partner. She bends at the waist and lifts her bottom up in the air. She crosses her arms on the back of the chair to support herself. He enters her from behind.

what she can do: Penetration will be deep, stimulating the front walls of the vagina and G-spot. She can adjust herself to hit these spots just right.

what he can do: As with all Doggy-Style variations, he mainly controls the movement, which can be a source of great pleasure for him, and this variation is by far one of the most exciting. He can hold on to her waist and control the rhythm, speed, and intensity of the thrusting. For her added pleasure, he can caress her clitoris and breasts with his hands.

BONUS!

This is a great position to transition to anal sex. Just go slowly, be gentle, and have plenty of lube on hand. Never go from anal sex to vaginal sex, however, because bacteria from the anus can cause a vaginal infection.

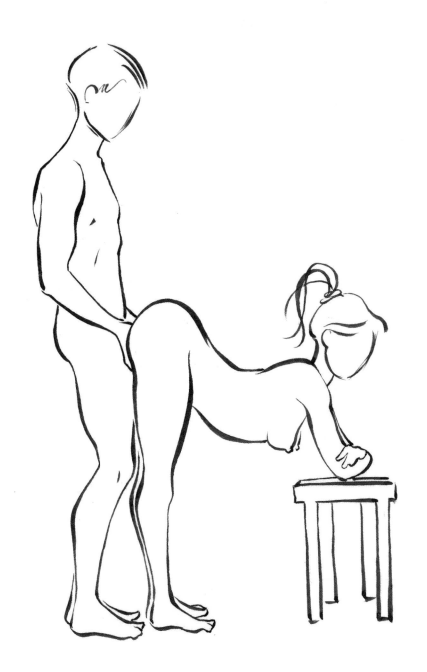

3.7 THE HOUND

Despite its name, which doesn't necessarily conjure up ideas of romance, the Hound is probably the most intimate when it comes to Doggy-Style variations. In this position, both partners are on their knees. She is on the inside, resting on her forearms. He is curled around her and enters her from behind.

what she can do: She can swivel her hips to find the right angle for the desired degree of penetration. She can reach back and caress his nipples or his testicles. She may turn her head to the side and initiate deep kissing.

what he can do: This position is great for slow, deep thrusting as well as quick, shallow thrusts. Start slow, and then go faster. Alternate between deep and shallow. In this variation there is more skin-to-skin contact, and breasts, nipples, clitoris, and anus are all within easy reach. He can nibble her ears, kiss her neck, or breathe dirty/sweet phrases down her back.

BONUS!

This is a great position to segue into after-sex spooning, when both are too tired and satiated to move into a more comfortable position.

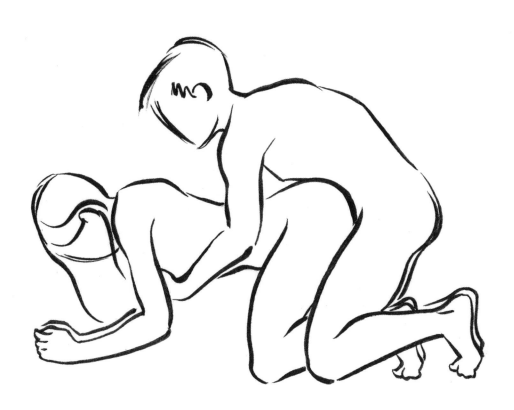

(3.8) THE **STANDING HOUND**

The Standing Hound is also known as the *Ben Dover* and is essentially Standing Doggy with her bending over at the waist. It's another great position to stretch out the legs or when lying down is not practical or possible (for example, in the shower, in the kitchen, or in an elevator). She bends over, hinging from the waist, and places her hands on the floor. She might also grab her ankles or her feet if she can't reach the floor. The bottom line is that she will need a way to find balance, which will allow for faster thrusting and a more enjoyable experience. When she is bent over, she pushes her pelvis back against him and he enters her from behind. She may need a little flexibility and some leg strength for this one, but it's possible to find some creative work-arounds.

what she can do: For variation she might try spreading her legs farther apart or bringing them closer together. This will change the angle and depth of penetration and may or may not work depending on their height differences. Bending her knees can help if she starts to get tired, or she may lean back onto him to rest her arms.

what he can do: He can bend his knees and lean back to change his angle of entry. He can also put his hands on her waist to help control the speed and depth of penetration. This position also affords him a great view and lets him reach around to stimulate her clitoris. He might try standing against a wall so she can push herself back onto him. He can bend at the knees while thrusting, go slow, and grind her G-spot.

> **BONUS!**
>
> He can reach down and grab her hair, which will be falling around her face. This can be a loving gesture or one of control and submission. You decide.

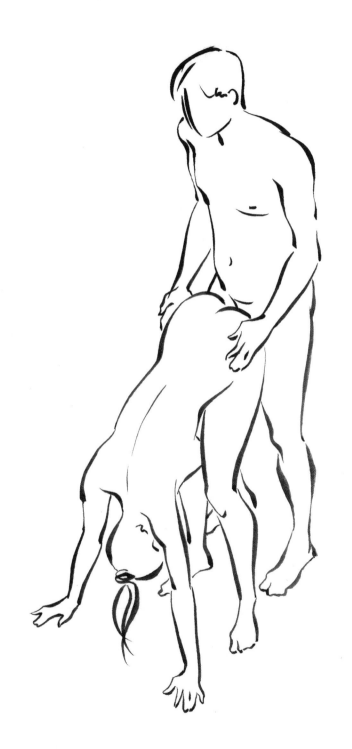

(3.9) THE HINGE

This variation of Doggy Style allows for more depth control. She is facing away from him in Doggy position, on all fours, while resting her weight on her forearms. From here she straightens her legs and spreads them wide apart. Standing, he approaches her from behind. He can hold her by the waist and pull up her legs so that he eventually grabs ahold of her ankles.

what she can do: She has some control of the movement in the Hinge. She moves herself forward and backward, shifting her weight to manage the angle and depth of penetration. She may also try leaning forward onto her elbows and thrusting her bottom back onto him or rest her legs on his thighs. A pillow beneath her forearms will soften the pressure.

what he can do: He has a nice view of her lovely ass. Once he gets into a good balanced position, with her lower half resting on his thighs, he can enjoy the view of her backside and of his penis going in and out of her.

> **BONUS!**
>
> This may be a more challenging position for them, as she is supporting her weight partially on her forearms and partially on his thighs. If he is strong, they may be able to see this position through to climax.

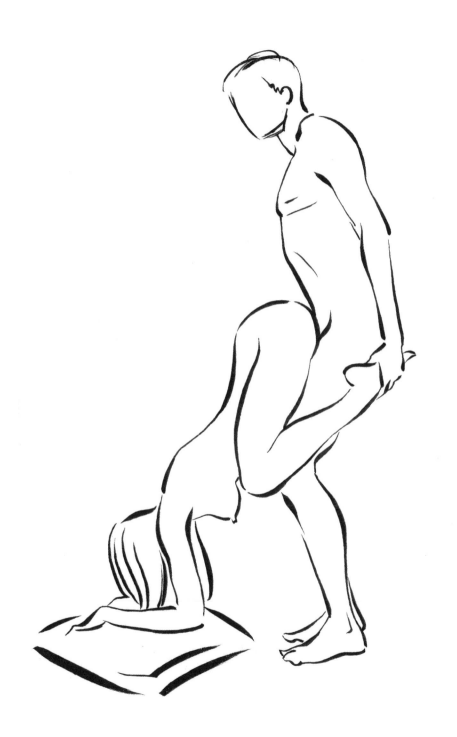

(3.10) BACKSEAT **DRIVER**

This is a seated variation of Doggy Style. It is a great one for doing on the floor, on the bed, or in the backseat of a car, hence the name. In this position, he is sitting on a bed or the floor with his legs straight out in front of him or bent at the knees. She bends her knees and lowers herself onto him, inside his lap, facing his feet. She will use her legs to bounce up and down on him.

what she can do: She is doing most of the work in this position, whether it is bouncing up and down or gyrating her hips for a slower circular grind, which will hit more erogenous zones inside and outside her vagina. Also, by leaning forward or backward, she can change the angle of penetration. She can put her hands on his thighs or hold on to something else for support.

what he can do: He can sit back and enjoy the ride or grab on to her hips and pull her down toward him with each stroke. Or he can grab her shoulders and pull her down in time with the thrusting. He can also place his hands under her butt to lift her up and down.

BONUS!

This is a great position to use for the Mile-High Club! While on an airplane, the man and woman wrangle themselves into one of those tiny bathrooms. He puts down the toilet seat and sits down and she backs up onto him and rests her hands on his thighs. Aside from him sitting on the toilet seat, neither person has to touch anything else in the bathroom (except the sink) and the remaining duration of the plane ride will be so much more enjoyable.

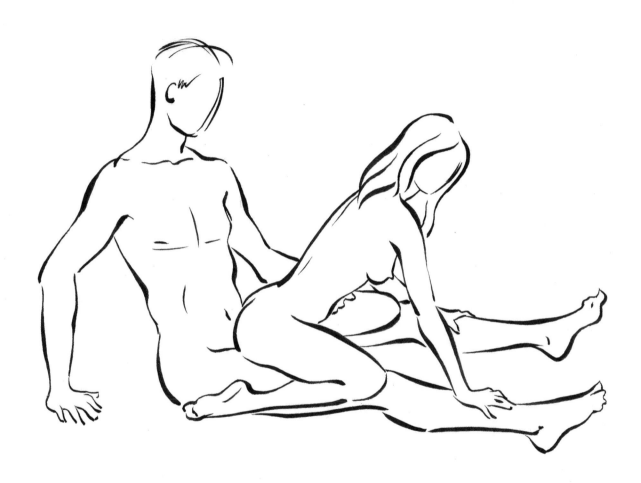

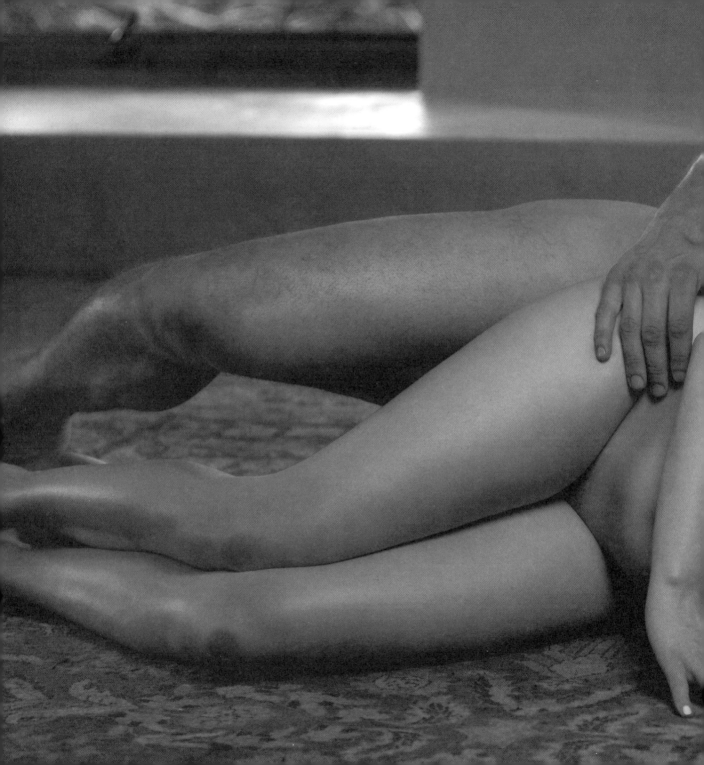

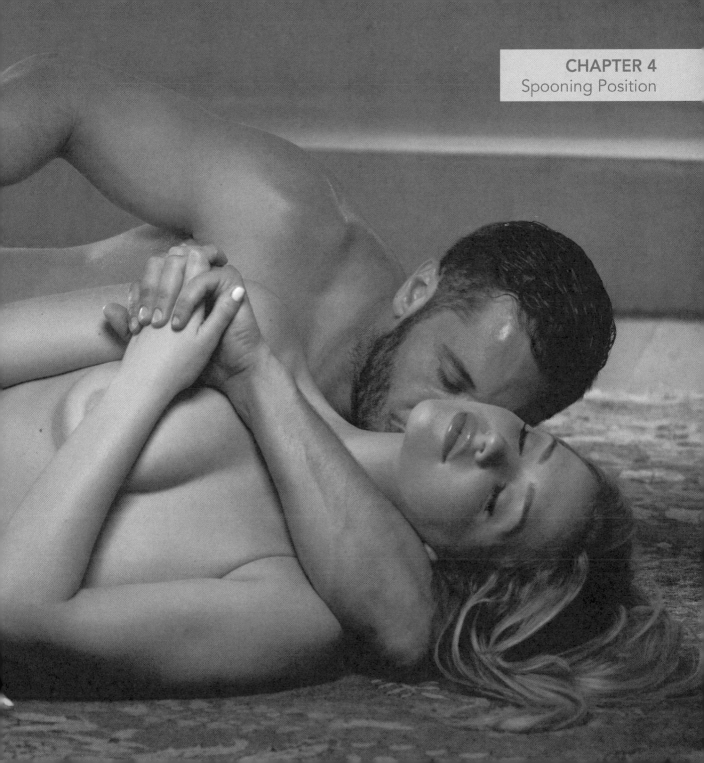

SPOONING POSITION

SPOONING IS A SEXUAL POSITION but also refers to a form of cuddling that is similar to hugging. The name refers to two spoons that, when positioned side by side, fit nicely together. The sexual version of spooning is a rear-entry position, with the woman on the inside and the man on the outside as the outer spoon. Because spooning is also a term for cuddling, this position has the potential for greater intimacy and body contact. On the other hand, there is little opportunity for eye contact and the close proximity prevents partners from seeing each other's bodies fully, limiting visual stimulation. Also, the angle may not be the best for intercourse because the penis may slip out easily.

However, this is a more relaxed position and is great for when the partners have just woken up or are fairly tired at the end of a long day. It is also a go-to position if the woman is pregnant. Especially during the last trimester, spooning is ideal because it does not put any pressure on the abdomen. The position is excellent for those with less body strength because it requires significantly less muscle power. Spooning is great in the backseat of a car, or on the couch right after your favorite movie has ended. Finally, spooning is not limited to two people, and is an easy position for three or even more.

How to Do It

In the Spooning position the man lies on his side with knees bent while she lies with her back pressed up against his body. Their legs can be resting side by side or on top of each other. From this position penetration is fairly straightforward; however, the partners may need to shift their bodies to get it right. For example, he might push himself up on his arms to get a better angle. She can lift her upper knee to allow for easier access. For partners who desire intimacy, this position maintains full-body contact and fosters safety and tenderness without bringing in significant imbalances of power. Both partners have control over the angle and depth of penetration.

benefits for her

Because her hands are free she can easily stimulate her clitoris with her fingers or a vibrator or reach down and massage his scrotum for his added pleasure. In addition, because the angle of his penis massages the front of her vagina, this is a great position for G-spot stimulation.

benefits for him

Because his hands are free, this is a fairly relaxing position and offers him the opportunity to caress her belly and breasts, kiss the back of her neck and ears, and reach down and stimulate her clitoris. He may also move his hands down and hold on to her hips for more control, or cup her buttocks in his palms to move her up and down.

HISTORICAL TIDBIT

It has long been a tradition for the Welsh to carve out spoons as a testament of their love for one another and as a symbol of togetherness. Spoons were even once used as engagement rings.

(4.1) SIDE **SADDLE**

This variation might be easier for thrusting and penetration. Once in the Spooning position, she moves her torso forward to give him better access for penetration.

what she can do: During penetration, she can keep her knees close together if it feels better. She might spread her legs slightly for easier access and control. From this position she is in control and can move up and down using her hands as support. She may also swivel her hips around or side to side to vary the motion and hit different erogenous zones.

what he can do: He can just lie back and enjoy the ride. From this position he has a better view of her body and his penis moving in and out of her vagina. He can use his hands to hold her hips for more control or to stimulate her breasts, nipples, and clitoris for added pleasure.

> **BONUS!**
>
> Because he is already lying back and relaxed, it is a great time to blindfold him to add to his delight.

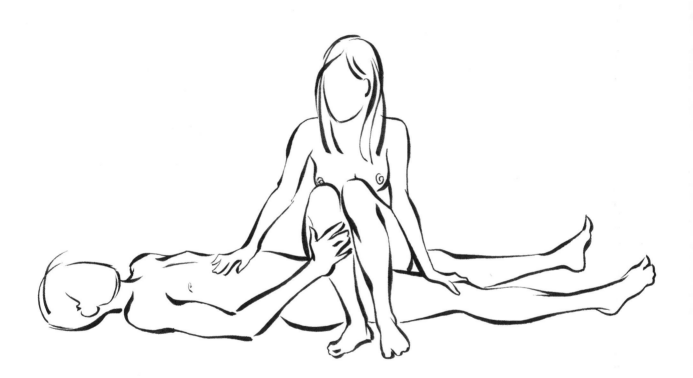

THE SPOON **AND FORK**

In this variation of spooning, often shortened to "spork," she rolls over and lies on her back. She raises the leg closest to him and can rest it on his shoulder or to the side. He positions himself between her legs at a 90-degree angle to her body, supporting himself with one arm behind his back, in a half-reclining position.

what she can do: She can lift her top leg even more to vary the angle and depth of penetration. Because her hands are free she can put them to good use: She can touch herself or reach down and hold the base of his penis as they thrust their hips together.

what he can do: He can lift up one of her legs to increase the depth of penetration. If he is more upright, this is also a good position for G-spot stimulation.

> **BONUS!**
>
> Put the blindfold on her for heightened sensory awareness and a feeling of complete surrender.

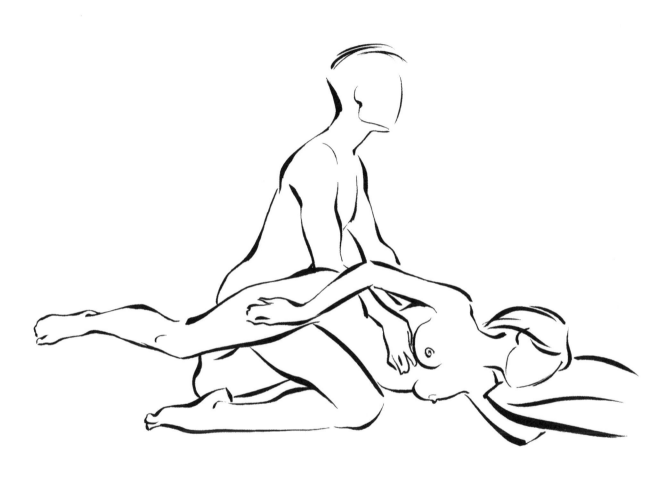

4.3 THE Y-SPLIT

In this position she stays lying on her side. Her legs are together. She may have a pillow under her head for extra support. He positions himself upright so he is kneeling, but his body is leaning over her body as he slides in between her legs. From here she can raise her top leg, giving him more access.

what she can do: In this variation, she has some control and can raise her hips to give him better access. She can control the angle of the thrusting by lifting or lowering her leg so that his penis hits her G-spot. The angle of his body may also allow for her to get some clitoral stimulation by rubbing her body against his. She can prop herself on her elbows or forearms to participate in the movement.

what he can do: One of his knees is between her legs, to make it easier for penetration. He should place his hands where he can get the support to help guide him. The angle of her legs and butt can give him deep access, and if her legs are close together it will provide more friction. He can hold her top leg and move it around to get better visuals and experiment with angles. If his hands are free, he can stimulate her breasts, nipples, or clitoris.

> **BONUS!**
>
> The entwined nature of this position fosters intimacy. Lovers can kick it up a notch by gazing deeply into each other's eyes, a technique the Kama Sutra recommends for melding as one during lovemaking.

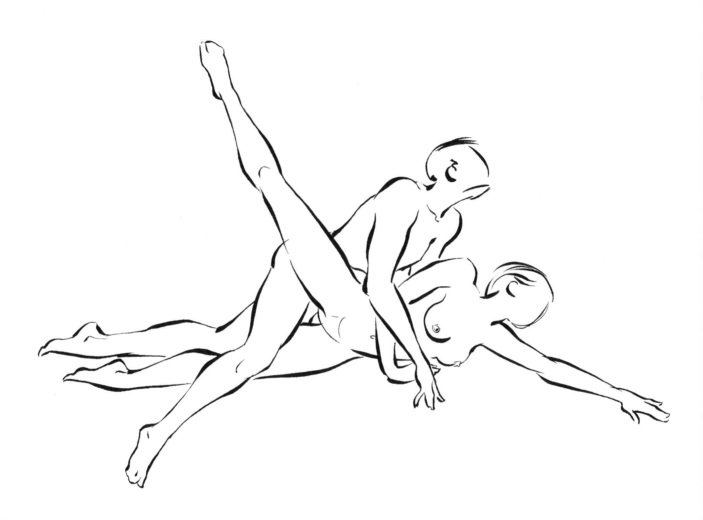

(4.4) THE CLOSE-UP

Originally termed the *anjou* by the Kama Sutra, the Close-Up is also known as the *curled angel* position. Still lying on their sides, the man spoons the woman from behind. The woman then curls her legs and brings her knees up toward her chest, allowing her partner to penetrate her from behind. The Close-Up is excellent for stimulating her G-spot, which often leads to explosive female orgasms.

what she can do: She can wrap her legs around the outside of his for a tighter squeeze. Because her hands are free, she can stimulate her clitoris, either with a hand or a vibrator. She can grind her hips to hit the various erogenous zones within her vagina.

Pregnant women may also find this position much more comfortable because it provides support for a growing baby bump. She can adjust her knees, bringing them up less or more depending on the size of her belly.

what he can do: This may be a somewhat easier version of spooning where his penis is less likely to slip out. To get the most out of this position, he can go slow, take his time, and build the intensity.

> **BONUS!**
>
> This position is great for anal sex with a finger, a toy, or a penis. With any anal play, it's important to go very slowly, use plenty of lube, and maintain good communication.

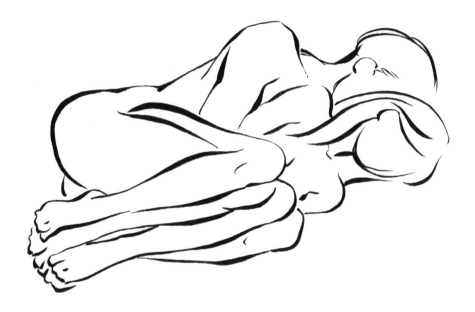

4.5 UPSIDE-DOWN **SPOONING**

This variation of spooning is also known as *poles apart*. This position may be awkward at first, and it may be a little tough to keep the penis inside the vagina. But it has the propensity to provide excellent G-spot stimulation and shallow penetration, which is perfect for women who don't like having their cervix bumped. Both partners lie on their sides, facing in the same direction. This is the part that is similar to traditional spooning. However, instead of lying head to head, one partner switches direction so they are now feet to head. He then enters her from behind. This position provides access to the legs and feet, which in other positions are typically neglected.

what she can do: Because it may feel like the penis keeps sliding out, she can shift the angle of her butt to make this a little easier. She can also reach behind and grab his butt to give the thrust some control and traction.

what he can do: He can try using gentle thrusts and hold on to her legs for greater support and deeper penetration.

> **BONUS!**
>
> Foot fetishists take note. Those who enjoy playing with feet, or having their feet rubbed and caressed, will find Upside-Down Spooning a particularly good fit. Specifically for him, her feet will be very close to his face, so he can use his hands and mouth to kiss, massage, and lick them.

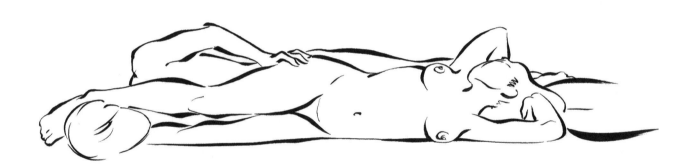

4.6 KNEELING **WHEELBARROW**

This position requires both partners to roll slightly until they are both on their knees. The man rolls over to be upright on his knees. The woman can still be on her side as in the Spooning position but lifts herself up on her forearm and lifts her bottom half up onto the knee on the same side. He kneels behind her. He can hold her hips to enter her while she either bends her other knee to give him better access or extends it back behind her. Placing pillows under the knees may provide more comfort in this position.

what she can do: Since her leg is up, this position is quite tiring for the woman and may be hard to maintain for a long period of time. Placing a sturdy pillow behind her to rest her leg on can help.

what he can do: From this position the man can stimulate her clitoris, breasts, or nipples. He can also hold her hips or waist to control the thrusting.

> **BONUS!**
>
> Some of these rear-entry positions may lead to quicker orgasms for him. Some things to do to extend the play include going slower and alternating deeper, harder thrusts with shorter, shallower thrusts. He can also try pulling out before climax and then reenter her for the feeling of penetration all over again. These techniques can make him last longer, feel more in control of his excitement, and give her the time and space to reach climax.

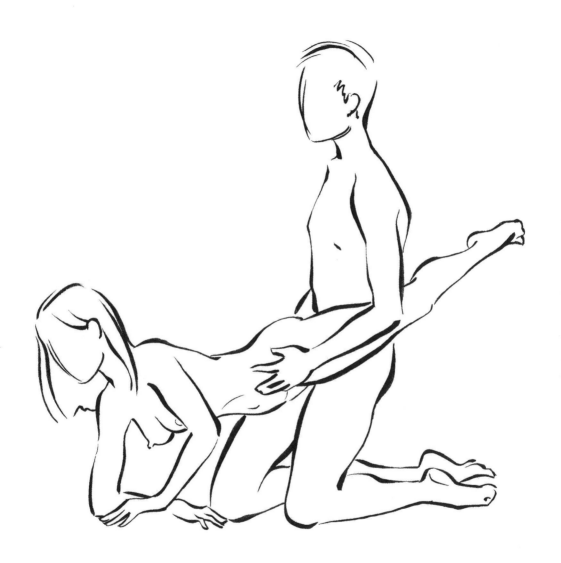

4.7 SIDEWAYS **SAMBA**

This position provides maximum penetration and deeper thrusting than can be achieved in the traditional form of spooning. The woman lies on her side with her back to him, similar to her position in traditional spooning. In this position, however, her legs are straight out in front of her at 90 degrees in the shape of an "L." He lies behind her on his side, still in the spoon position. He may raise himself up onto his hands, placing his outer hand on the other side of her body next to her chest to assist with maneuvering into penetration.

what she can do: She can shift her hips around to find what feels best for her and to hit different spots inside the vagina. She can keep her legs closed for a feeling of tighter penetration while also keeping the thrusts shallow, or arch her back and spread her legs to increase the depth of the thrusts.

what he can do: Penetration and thrusting are mostly under his control. Because of the angle, he may also do more intense thrusting. The slippery angle of this variation can sometimes cause his penis to slip out. He can use this to his advantage, to prolong orgasm and build on the excitement for more intense pleasure.

BONUS!

There's nothing like a little restraint to bring a naughty edge to sex. With her consent, he can bind her legs together around the ankles using a tie, a strap from a bathrobe, or one of her scarves. This will keep her legs together, a key to this position, and add to the power play between the couple.

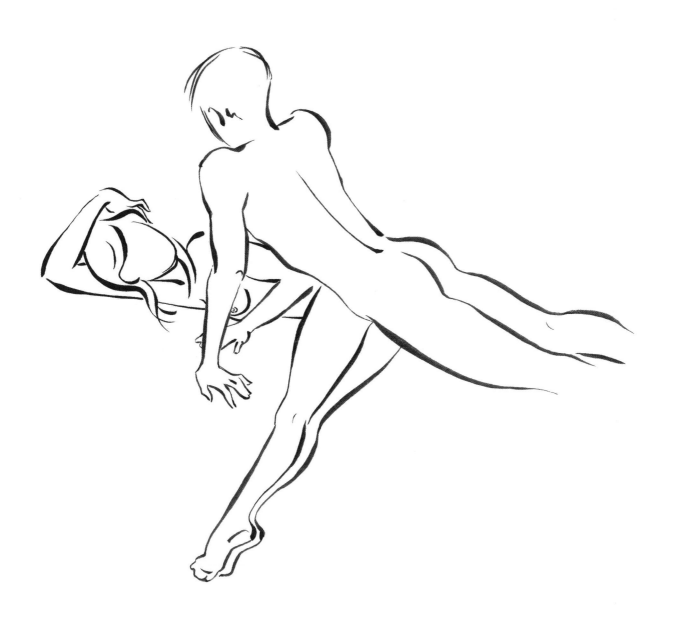

(4.8) THE **SIDEKICK**

This is another variation of spooning in which the woman gets to relinquish some control while also experiencing deep penetration and G-spot stimulation. The couple starts by lying down on their sides in the original Spooning position. The man then rolls himself up onto his knees so that he is kneeling behind her, facing the back of her head. He then slides one knee in between her legs, spreading her legs apart for better access so that he may enter her.

what she can do: She may move her top leg forward to give herself better balance and more control while also giving him a better view. This action also helps her control some of the depth and motion of the thrusts.

what he can do: Going slow and steady to build up some intensity works great in this position. Because of the positioning of her legs and the angle of her vagina, this variation may make it harder for him to enter her initially, but ultimately it could be the perfect angle to stimulate her G-spot. Building up speed, then pulling the penis out and reentering her is also a great way to prolong arousal for more intense orgasms. He may hold on to her hips as he thrusts, or place his hands on the bed or on her back.

> **BONUS!**
>
> With his thigh between her legs she has the perfect excuse to engage in a little high school–style dry humping—only this time not so dry! Put a little lube on his thigh and the friction will feel even better.

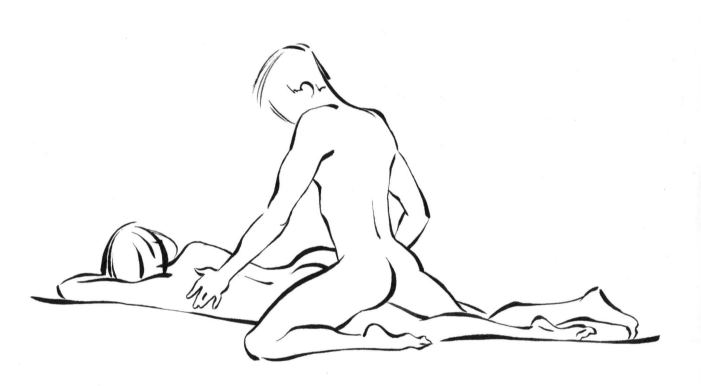

4.9 THE **CRISSCROSS**

This variation of spooning is great for shallow grinding, arousing visuals, and better control. Similar to the Spooning position, the woman starts by lying on her side, with her arms above her head or beside her head in a crisscross. The man also lies on his side but his body is perpendicular to hers.

what she can do: She can raise her top leg so he may slide in between her thighs. She can control the depth and intensity of the penetration by shifting her torso to the left or right, whichever feels best for her. She may swivel her hips as well. If she needs a little more action, her hands are free to stimulate her clitoris, nipples, or breasts.

what he can do: He can hold on to her shoulders to assist with penetration and thrusting. The perpendicular angle lets him have some great visuals of his penis going in and out. The thrusting from this angle can be shallow, focusing on her G-spot, or deeper, for intense pleasure.

> **BONUS!**
>
> There is little eye contact and skin-to-skin intimacy in this position, but couples can use that to their advantage. This is a perfect time to indulge in private fantasies or role-play sex with a stranger.

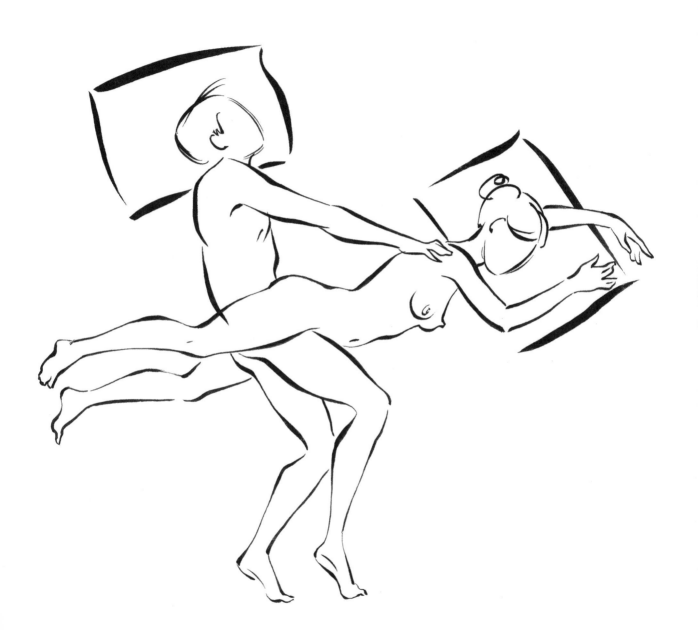

(4.10) AFTERNOON **DELIGHT**

Afternoon Delight is a great position for those who need a break from intense sex or are just feeling a bit lazy, aroused but lacking energy. It also allows for more skin-to-skin contact, and both can enjoy the intimacy of gazing into each other's eyes. He lies on his side, as if about to spoon her, and she lies at a right angle to him, on her back with her knees bent. She slides her legs up over his hip, so that the backs of her knees are resting on his hip.

what she can do: Her hands are free to caress her clitoris, breasts, and nipples, and if she is close enough, she can reach over to stimulate his testicles or perineum. She can raise her hips to gain control of the thrusting and to increase the intensity. She can lift and spread her legs to give him a better view.

what he can do: He can caress her nipples or clitoris or relax and watch her pleasure herself, which can be highly arousing.

> **BONUS!**
>
> This position causes little stress or strain and may be ideal for partners with extreme height differences, injuries, or health issues where physical exertion is a concern.

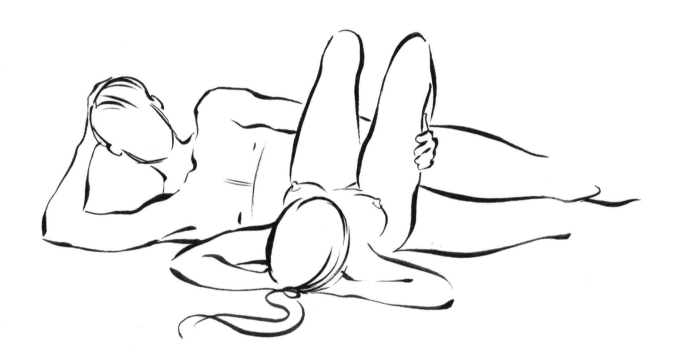

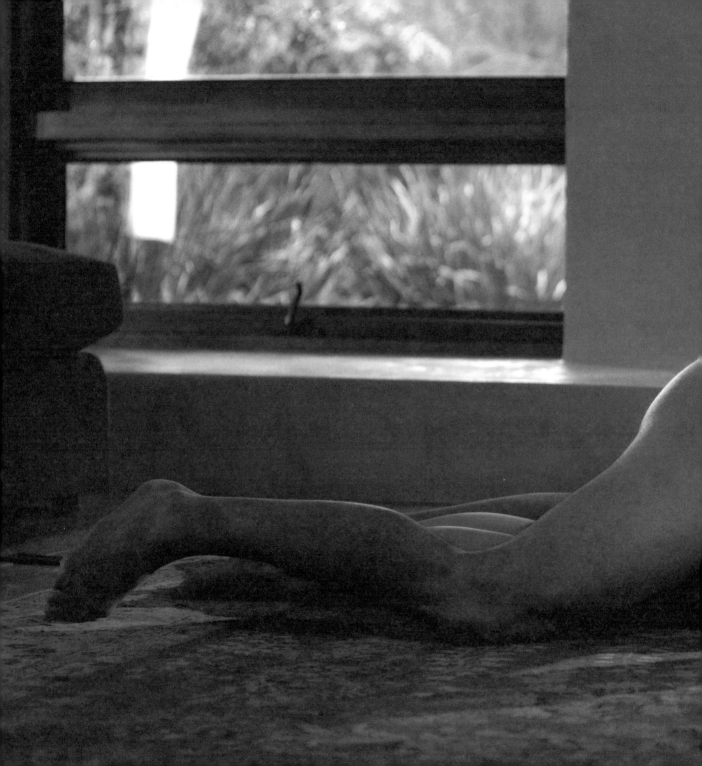

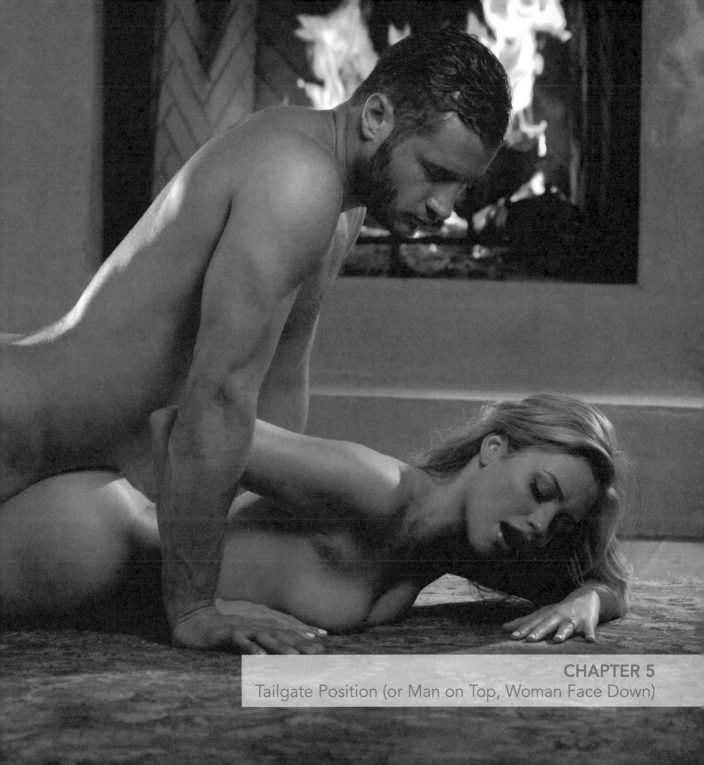

CHAPTER 5
Tailgate Position (or Man on Top, Woman Face Down)

TAILGATE POSITION
(OR MAN ON TOP, WOMAN FACE DOWN)

THIS CLASSIC POSITION WHERE THE MAN IS ON TOP and the woman is face down is known as the Tailgate and is a form of rear entry. For many women, this position can stimulate the G-spot or the A-spot, an erogenous zone inside her vagina, on the anterior wall, a little higher up than the G-spot. Many women find this area very sensitive. Even though it does not offer a lot of eye contact, this position still provides intimacy because his body is on top of hers and there is lots of skin-to-skin connection. This position is great for seduction and building arousal, as a warm-up to intercourse, and can be a sexy way for a man to wake up his bed partner in the morning.

How to Do It

The woman lies face down on her stomach and the man lies down on her. The man penetrates her from behind. For some couples it may be better for him to be on his knees, placing them on each side of her legs, thus pushing her legs together. This may prevent his penis from slipping out.

benefits for her

This might be a position that is best for morning sex, when she is still tired—that is, if she is not sleeping. Because sex and sleep don't always mix, partners who enjoy "sleepy-time sex" should discuss it with each other prior to making any sudden moves. Sleepy-time sex can be enjoyable if precious sleep is not being disrupted. Or she may just act like she is sleeping. The man can creep up from behind. This can bring a heightened sense of surrender for her and intensify the sense of control for him. She can grab on to the bedposts for more traction and to further intensify the sense of surrender/domination.

benefits for him

Starting slow will build heat. This can be a good way to initiate sex if she is already in bed and lying on her stomach. He can start by lying on top of the sheets while she is underneath and talk dirty into her ear to build arousal.

> **BONUS**
>
> This is an excellent position for giving her a back massage that she will love. He should start at her shoulders and work his way down her back to her butt and thighs. Harder and stronger massages are great for working those back muscles and inspiring relaxation but this might put her right back to sleep. Light massages, on the other hand, can arouse her most subtle erogenous zones. The spine is chockfull of nerve endings, which extend out to her lower back, hips, and inner and outer thighs, and when very lightly stimulated (i.e., with a feather or your tongue) will send the chill right back down to her pelvis area.

5.1 THE **SLEEPING BEAUTY**

In the Sleeping Beauty variation, she may be sleeping lightly; however, she will probably need to be somewhat awake to get the most out of this variation. Her bottom is pushed up in the air, like a small hump, and her legs are spread slightly apart, for easier access for him and more opportunities for self-exploration for her. He lies on top of her, with his bottom half between her legs, and props his top half up on his hands. He then enters her from behind.

what she can do: If penetration proves difficult, she can try placing a pillow under her stomach or pelvis. In this position, she can reach underneath and stimulate herself, or press herself against a vibrator or pillow. She can also push her bottom up higher to give him better access and allow for deeper penetration; lowering her bottom to the bed will create more shallow penetration. Pushing herself up onto her arms might also be a more comfortable position for her.

what he can do: He has control of the thrusting. He can go slowly in the beginning to get the right motion and position. His hands can be on the bed, supporting him. If he lies down on her, he will have less control. Dirty talk is a great way to add some excitement to this position.

> **BONUS!**
>
> This position is great for anal intercourse as well.

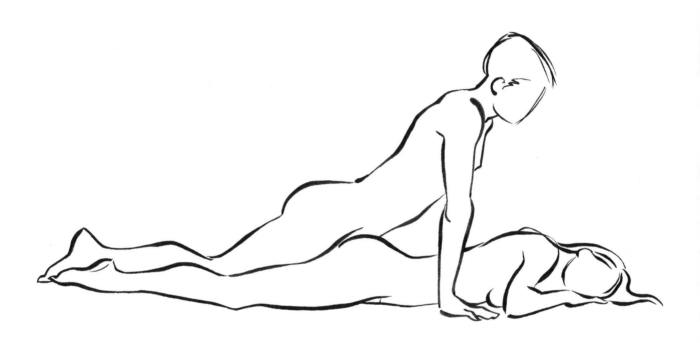

5.2 HIT THE **SPOT**

As the name suggests, this position is perfect for hitting her G-spot and other erogenous zones inside her vagina. The woman lies on her stomach with her hips turned to one side and her legs bent. The man kneels between her legs and leans forward with his arms on each side of her.

what she can do: This position can hit her G-spot, A-spot, or other erogenous zones, and she can squirm her butt and change the angle of her hips to hit them all.

what he can do: He can remain upright and use his body strength to thrust, or he can place his hands on the bed to gain control of the action. Pushing his thigh underneath her will slide her legs up higher.

> **BONUS!**
>
> Because he has all the control in this position, he can tease her by playing up his power: pulling her hair—gently—or holding her hands behind her back. The sense that she is being objectified can be intensely arousing for her, while he can enjoy the feeling of her losing complete control. Be sure to check in with her to make sure she likes it.

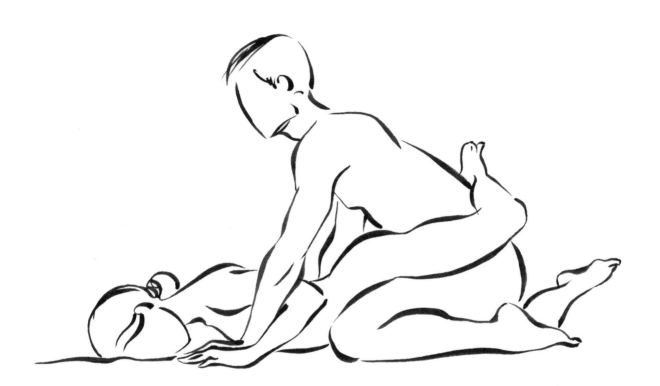

(5.3) THE PERCH

The couple can roll themselves upright and use a chair in this rear-entry variation called the Perch. The man pulls her up off the bed, right onto a chair, stool, or perch, and sits her in his lap. He can try this with his penis still inside her, which can be an exciting challenge.

what she can do: She will get a lot more action on the front part of her vagina in this position, plus she will have a little more control. She can use her legs for leverage to go up and down on his penis, swivel her hips in circles, or rock back and forth. She can lean back to give him more access to her clitoris and breasts, or lean forward to give him a good view of her ass.

what he can do: He can hold her hips to get more control and move her up and down. Or, if she is in control of the motion, he can reach forward and stimulate her clitoris, breasts, and nipples.

> **BONUS!**
>
> Although there is potential for clitoral orgasm in this position, it is also ripe for her to have a joint clitoral/G-spot orgasm. The key is finding the right spot inside the vagina and building up the intensity and speed.

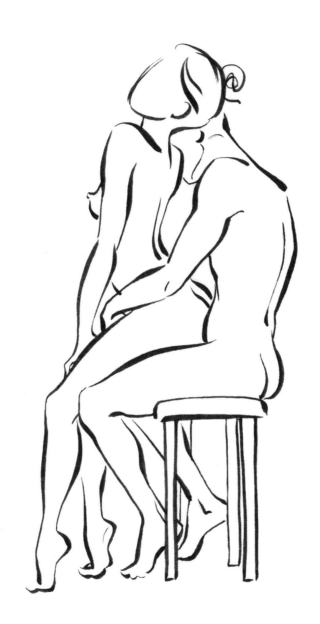

5.4 THE **LANDSLIDE**

Depending on the angle of his erect penis, the Landslide may pose a challenge for direct penetration, but with a little effort this can stimulate her G-spot, as it lends itself to more shallow access. She lies down on her stomach. Her head and shoulders are propped up on her forearms and her legs are straight behind her and slightly apart. He sits right behind her butt, with his legs in front of him, and leans back onto his hands. When he finds the perfect angle for penetration, she brings her legs together for a tight fit.

what she can do: She has little control in this position, with the exception of being able to close her legs to provide a little friction. As with many of the rear-entry positions, she may find a submissive position arousing.

what he can do: He may need to shift around to get that perfect fit, but once he finds it he can control the thrusting using his arms as leverage. He has a great view of going in and out of her vagina and may get a good view of her vulva.

> ### BONUS!
>
> Consensual BDSM (bondage, domination, and sadomasochism) can be a great way to add excitement to a relationship, and the thrill of doing something edgy and a bit naughty can be a real turn-on. This is a great position to incorporate some light BDSM because she is already in a very submissive posture. Mutual trust is important in this type of play, as is having a "safe word" that will halt the action as soon as anyone gets uncomfortable.

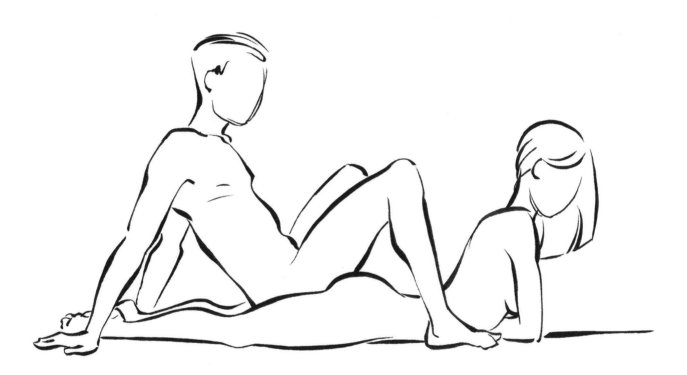

(5.5) THE SPHINX

The Sphinx conjures up visions of a mythical royal creature, half-lion and half-human, and in many ways the Sphinx sex position just might live up to the name. The woman lies on her belly. Her head is up, with her upper body weight supported by her forearms. One of her legs can be bent out to the side, while the other is outstretched behind her. Here she looks similar to the great Egyptian statue. He is on top and behind her, supporting his weight on his arms. His legs can be bent or stretched out behind him.

what she can do: The angle of her bottom, coupled with the pressure of his body on her pelvis, will stimulate her vulva. She can make sure her clitoris is rubbing against the bed while his penis is hitting her G-spot, leading to a powerful blended clitoral and G-spot orgasm.

what he can do: Alternating the thrusting from slow and deep to quick and shallow can tease her and give him a sense of control. Taking breaks from intense thrusting is really the key when it comes to building up arousal for an intense climax.

> **BONUS!**
>
> Because partners can't see each other's faces or make eye contact, communication becomes especially important in rear-entry positions. Letting it out verbally is sometimes more arousing than the physical act itself.

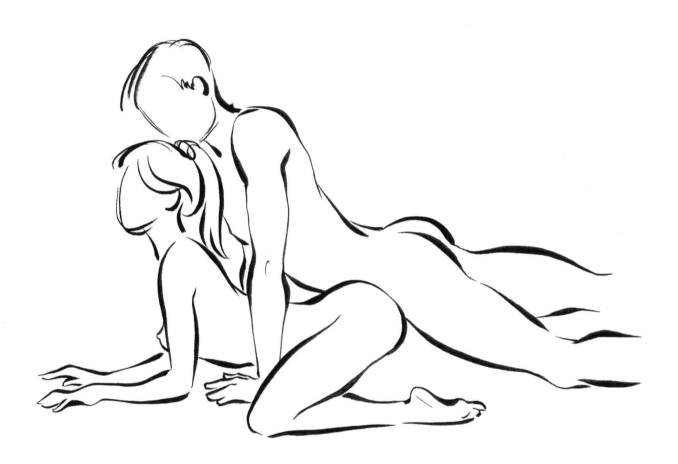

(5.6) THE Y-CURVE

This position works if the couple is already in the Tailgate position but her head is facing the bottom of the bed. The couple scoots down so her top half slides off the bed. Her head and torso reach down toward the ground, while she uses her hands to support her head. His legs are straight in between hers.

what she can do: She can rotate or swivel her hips to get a better angle. His weight on her might be an issue, which prevents her from having much flexibility in this position. This variation may be easier for women with strong core muscles.

what he can do: He can place his hands on her buttocks for support, or he can hold on to her hips. He will get more thrusting force if he arches his back.

BONUS!

This might be the least intimate and sexually submissive position of them all, but that can be a good thing! Not only is he having his way with her, but also he can't even see her face or the top half of her body. It is almost like a faceless being to do with as he wishes. If she enjoys this sense of being objectified, she can play it up however she likes.

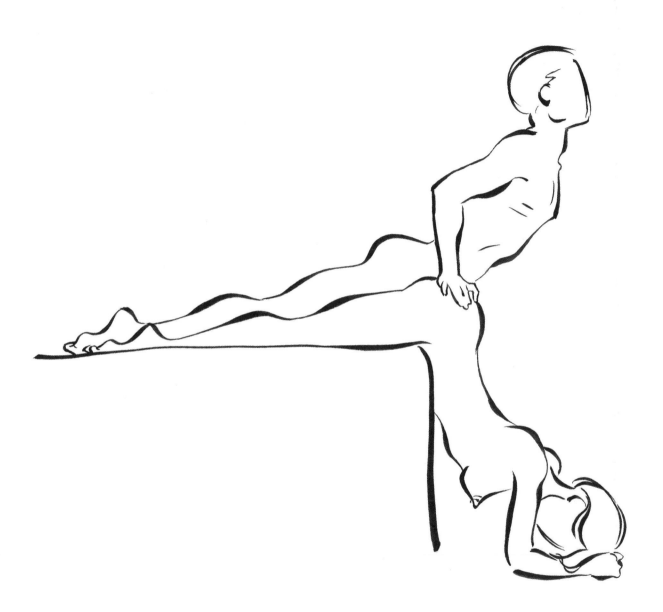

5.7 THE **APPROACHING TIGER**

This variation can bring some closeness and intimacy back into play if staying in a rear-entry position is desired. She lies face down on the bed, her knees slightly bent and hips slightly raised. Having a pillow under her belly raises the angle of her hips. He enters from behind and props himself up on his arms for support. The pillow is key in this variation. It brings her body closer to his, making for more skin-to-skin contact, and this angle is great for direct penetration with very little chance of his penis slipping out. The snug fit of this position can make heavy thrusting enjoyable.

what she can do: She can rock back and forth on the pillow to find the angle that suits her.

what he can do: He can place his legs outside of hers for an even snugger fit.

> ### BONUS!
>
> A bullet vibe is a great toy for adding extra stimulation without the use of hands. She can slip it between her labia as she lies on the pillow or place it on the pillow and grind against it. Some bullets come with remote-control operation for the ultimate in power and submission fantasies.

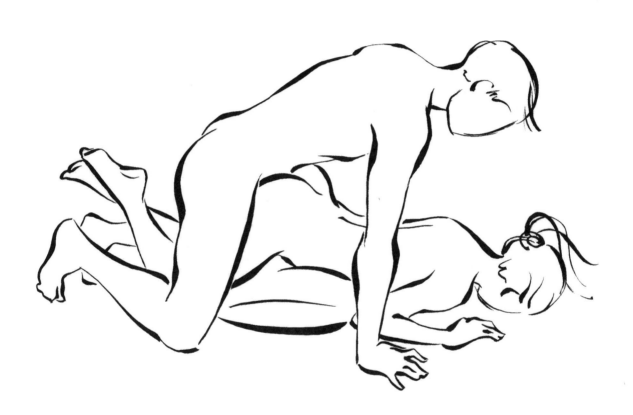

5.8 THE CAMELBACK

In the Camelback variation of Tailgate, the woman is on her knees, face down, with her hips raised in the air. She is bent forward from the waist down at an angle of about 45 degrees and her arms are splayed out to each side of her head a few inches past her shoulders. She uses her arms for support. He enters her from behind.

what she can do: If she needs to find more comfortable variations within the Camelback, she can rest her weight on her forearms. Arching her back might also make it easier for him to enter her. She can shift her hips around to find an angle that hits her G-spot.

what he can do: He will love this position for its excellent view of her backside and his penis going in and out of her. He can also control the motion by holding on to her hips. The position may be too direct an angle for her, so he should beware of hitting her cervix too hard. He can opt for shorter, shallower thrusts if she is uncomfortable with the depth of penetration.

> **BONUS!**
>
> Because this position leaves little opportunity for stimulating her breasts and clitoris, she might need some extra help in the way of lubrication. It is always a good idea to have some water-based or silicone-based lubrication on hand. There are many different varieties and brands, so experimenting with what works best is key.

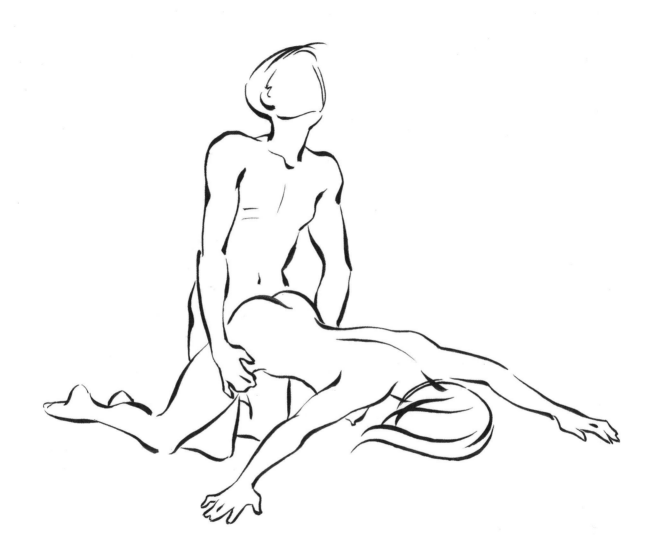

(5.9) THE **FLYING CIRCUS**

For those who really want to break out of their shell and try something a bit more daring, the Flying Circus might be just the thing. This position requires a little more upper body strength on his part, and she will need to have a lot of trust in his abilities. She must have some stamina as well to be able to maintain this position with him. Lying on the bed in a rear-entry position, he moves into a standing position holding on to her body, which is straight with her legs outstretched in back. It might look as though she is flying. Once they are in a fairly comfortable and stable position, thrusting can begin.

what she can do: She can reach back and hold on to his upper arms.

what he can do: Slow and steady wins the race in this position, which means long, slow thrusts will be easier to maintain. Depending on his strength, he may be able to carry her with him as he leaves the bed. If not, after he is upright, he can enter her and then lift her off the bed.

> **BONUS!**
>
> This position conjures up images of mad passion in the form of loud, unbridled sex. Letting it out in a noisy manner might also add to the fun and free-spirited nature of this position.

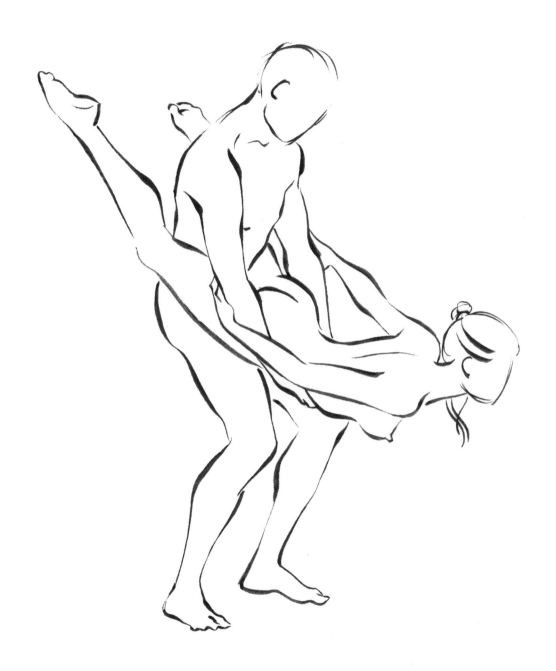

(5.10) POLES **APART**

To get into the Poles Apart variation of the Tailgate position, she rolls onto her side, with her back to him, and turns 180 degrees so her feet are near his head. Or they can slide down together so they meet closer in the middle. He will have easy access to her hips and thighs and can easily slide his penis into her. Even though their heads and faces are poles apart, they are curled forward, and the bend in their bodies allows for more eye contact than any of the other rear-entry positions. This is an excellent position to see each other's facial expressions of arousal, excitement, and orgasm. There is also quite a bit of skin-to-skin contact in this position.

what she can do: She can swing her legs over his hips to get into a more comfortable position with greater access to her vagina.

what he can do: He can grab her by her thighs and hips to maneuver into a good position for penetration. He can lavish attention on her inner and outer thighs.

BONUS!

This variation is excellent for him to initiate oral sex on her. Depending on their heights (for shorter torsos), his face may be close to her vagina. He may also pull out to give himself more room. In much the same vein, he has excellent access to her clitoris and vulva, which makes this rear-entry position a favorite among women.

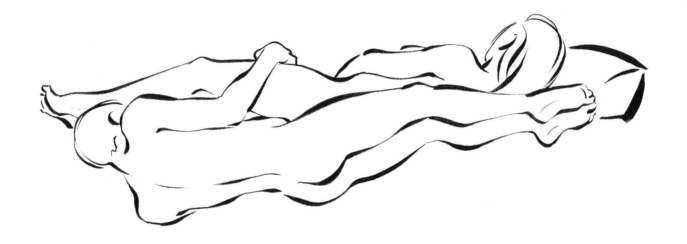

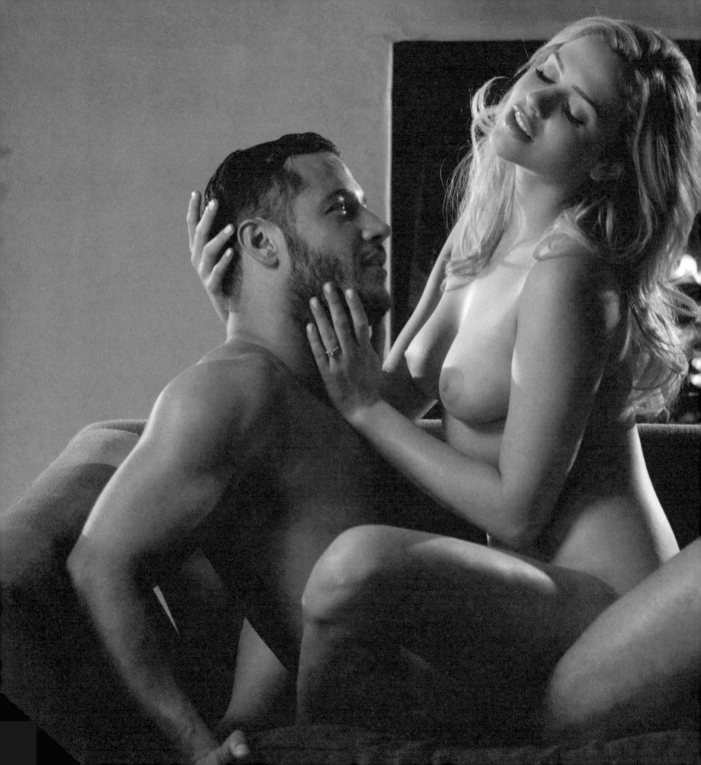

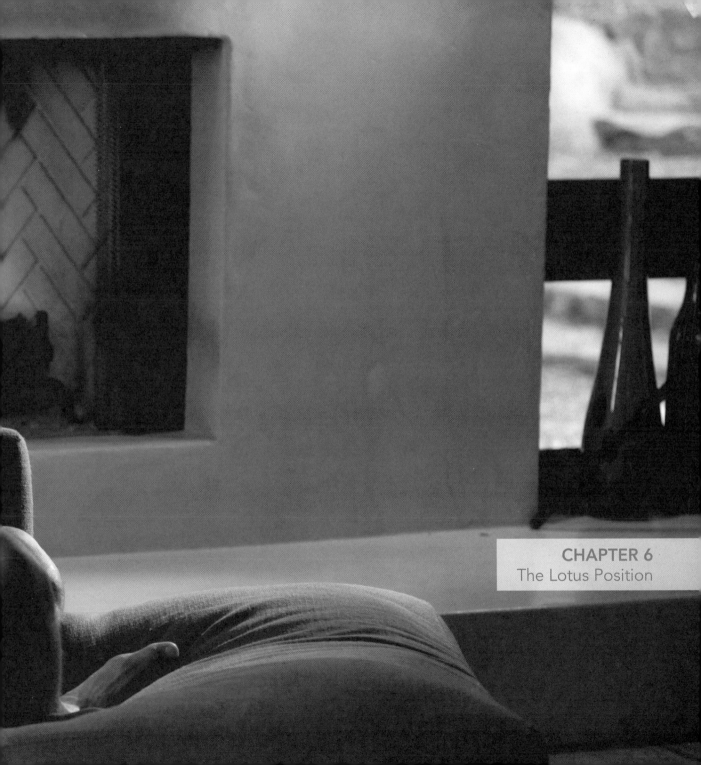

CHAPTER 6
The Lotus Position

THE LOTUS POSITION

THE LOTUS POSITION has the potential to build a lot of intimacy between a man and a woman. This position brings the couple face to face and eye to eye, with a lot of skin contact. The man and woman are mirroring one another and are entwined together, both in a similar position. Based on the traditional teachings of the *Kama Sutra*, the Lotus Position inspires calm and relaxation, which are key to mastering the art of any classic sex position.

How to Do It

First the man sits cross-legged on the bed or on the floor. She then sits on him, facing him, with her legs wrapped around his waist. Her legs can dangle a little bit off the bed as well, if there is room. In this position the man is grounded, while she floats more freely above him. The position may require the man to have a certain amount of flexibility and strength. He should be able to hold her up by the hips to control penetration and thrusting.

She can wrap her arms around him and hold tight, or she can rest her arms on his shoulders and use him to push herself up and down during thrusting. She has the option of being in control or letting him do the work. She can also lean back and put her hands on the bed, pushing her pelvis toward him to give him better access, a more direct view, and easier insertion. With her hands behind her, she can rotate her hips in circles to get a different kind of penetration.

benefits for both

If both partners are flexible, this can be a more prolonged position. The couple can intensify the intimacy with deep kissing; gazing into each other's eyes; nibbling each other's ears, neck, throat, and chest; and stimulating each other's nipples. However, the position may be more difficult to get into or sustain for those with hip, knee, or lower back stress.

While many positions highlight either strong feminine or alpha masculine roles, this one embraces harmony and equality. Both have an equal view of the action and can take charge of the thrusting and penetration either simultaneously or by alternating.

Deep relaxation can help build flexibility and sustain the position. Relaxation also aids orgasm. If orgasm is the desired goal, breathing deeply together in a meditative style can heighten sensation and enhance responsiveness. This position encourages the couple to engage all of their senses and stay present in the moment, which can lead to intense orgasm.

HISTORICAL TIDBIT

The lotus pose originated in the ancient Hindu and Buddhist traditions, in India and in China, as the preferred posture for sitting meditation and encourages long, deep, and relaxed breathing. The position is believed to bring about well-being, stability, and a sense of calm. A lotus pattern may also be created with the hands.to invite insight, wellness, and peace of mind.

6.1 LAP DANCE **SQUARED**

This variation of the Lotus position invites creative, wild, and flirty fun. A lap dance is a well-known dance that a woman can do for a man to arouse, tease, and play, and is often seen in strip clubs, but it is definitely not limited to them. Most men find that a lap dance is intense foreplay. Getting in the position is much the same as the Lotus. It's what the couple does beforehand that gets this variation going.

what she can do: The woman can engage all of the man's senses. She can put on some sultry, sexy dance music and wear something sensual, such as lingerie. Or she can wear her regular clothes and have sexy lingerie underneath, revealing the lingerie with a striptease first. The key to a lap dance is holding eye contact with him. While the eyes are locked in, she can dance herself toward him, gyrating her hips and shoulders as she slowly makes her way across the room. The key here is the visuals: He gets to watch her confident, sexy body. When she is ready she can climb into his lap, wrap her arms around his neck, and have a make-out session. Then, when both are ready, let the thrusting begin.

what he can do: He can hold on to her hips and squeeze her ass as she sits on his lap. He can continue intense eye contact to show that he is appreciating her efforts. And he can enjoy the show she is putting on for him and respond with approval and acceptance.

> **BONUS!**
>
> It's no mystery that a confident woman or man is sexy. Partners can take turns enacting the seductive ritual this position invites. It will not only make sex more fun but will also build a stronger, more vibrant connection for all sex play.

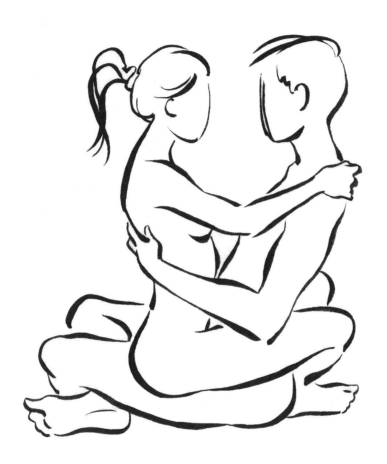

6.2 SPLITTING THE **BAMBOO**

This variation requires a little flexibility. From the Lotus position, she lies back on the bed, bends one leg, and extends the other leg over his shoulder. He kneels and straddles her bent leg.

what she can do: Because her hands are free, she can stimulate herself. She can also arch her back and tilt her pelvis to encourage G-spot stimulation.

what he can do: He can use a free hand to touch her and caress the leg that is resting on his shoulder. He can hold on to her upstretched thigh or her hips to push her up and down on him.

BONUS!

Both partners have a clear view of each other's faces and can watch each other's responses and expressions. This builds intimacy and heightens arousal.

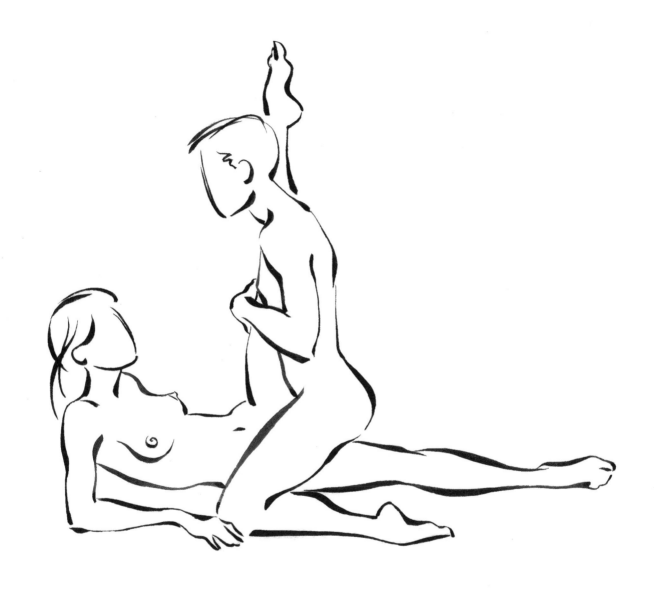

6.3 THE GLOWING **JUNIPER**

This intimate and erotic variation is easy to move into from the Lotus position. From his kneeling or sitting position, he straightens his legs out. From her position on his lap, she simply leans back and lies down between his legs. Or she can get into this position while straddling him as he is sitting. Her knees can be bent.

what she can do: She can squeeze her legs around his midsection to engage her pelvic floor muscles and create a snugger fit.

what he can do: He can place his hands under her bottom or under her back to move her body down onto him and slide inside her. This way, he can maneuver her body to control the thrusting. If his hands are free, this angle is great for stimulating her clitoris, breasts, and nipples.

> **BONUS!**
>
> This variation is good for hitting her G-spot and stimulating her clitoris simultaneously. Women can have blended orgasms stemming from this combination, which can mean a longer, more powerful, and more intense climax.

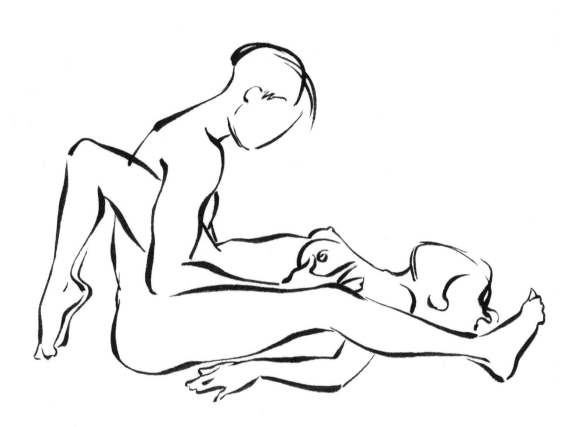

(6.4) ROW HIS **BOAT**

This variation of the Lotus allows him to relax a little bit while giving her more control, or they can share the efforts. There is also a good amount of eye contact in this position. He sits in an armchair, possibly reclining. She squats on his lap. Her legs are on the armrests to hold her in place for the squat. She can place her hands on his shoulders or on the top of the chair for support. She should be able to push herself up and down on his penis.

what she can do: This is another great position for her to give him a show. If she leans back he will be able to see his penis moving in and out of her vagina as well as her exposed vulva. She can gyrate her hips around in circles to stimulate various erogenous zones inside her vagina.

what he can do: Because this variation requires a little more leg strength on her part, he can support her weight by grabbing her hips and pulling her down onto him. Or, if she is doing all the work, he can stimulate her clitoris or nipples.

> **BONUS!**
>
> This position requires a chair that can recline and has arms . . . does that sound like an office chair? If he is working late and the office is empty, she can surprise him by bringing in dinner and then treating him to dessert.

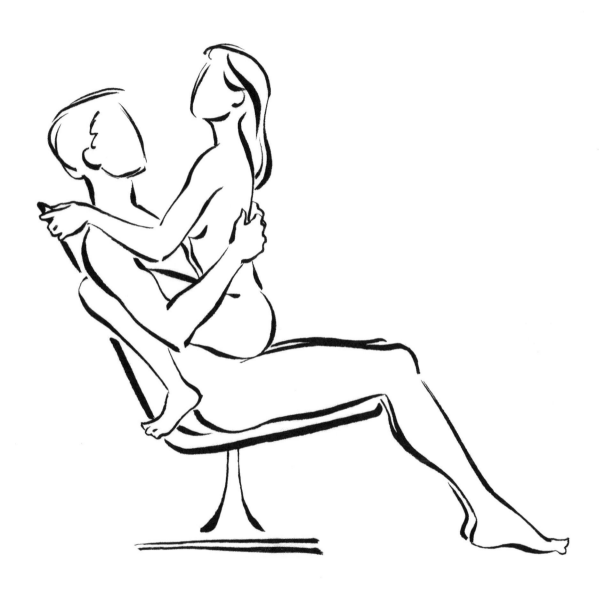

6.5 THE **KNEELING LOTUS**

This variation is very similar to the original Lotus position with one slight yet noticeable difference. Just as the name suggests, he kneels on the bed instead of sitting with his legs crossed. She sits down on him, facing him and straddling him, and wraps her legs around his torso, or she can bend her knees and place them on the bed.

what she can do: She can wrap her arms around his neck and shoulders to make it easier to move up and down or around in circles.

what he can do: He can hold her lower back during penetration and grab her ass to bring her closer to him.

BONUS!

Much like the original Lotus, there is a lot of equality in this position. Together they can find a groove that works for them. The closeness of this position allows for prolonged eye contact and kissing. There is a lot of room to get more sensual in this position and feel more connected.

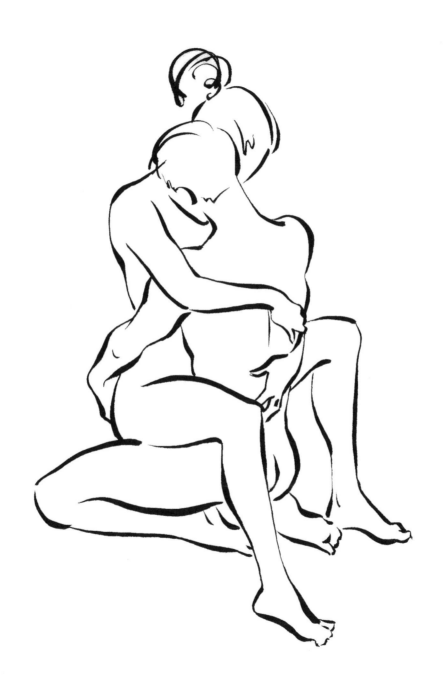

6.6 THE **RECLINING LOTUS**

She can put her flexibility to the test in the Reclining Lotus. To get into this position from the sitting Lotus, she simply keeps her legs crossed and lies back. He lies on top of her legs and enters her from there. He can rest his weight on his arms and knees to put less of his body weight on her.

what she can do: If she is flexible, her thighs and hips will get a nice stretch, but women who have tight hips or thighs may have difficulty in this position. She can uncross her legs for a slightly easier pose.

what he can do: He will have excellent access to and visuals of her vulva and clitoris. Since he is above her, and they are face to face, there is also opportunity for eye contact and kissing, the keys to intimacy.

> **BONUS!**
>
> Her crossed legs will prevent him from putting his full weight on her abdomen. This might be a good position for early pregnancy, when she may feel the need to protect the baby growing inside her. Or, if she has her period and is experiencing cramps, this might be a good option for avoiding too much pressure on the belly.

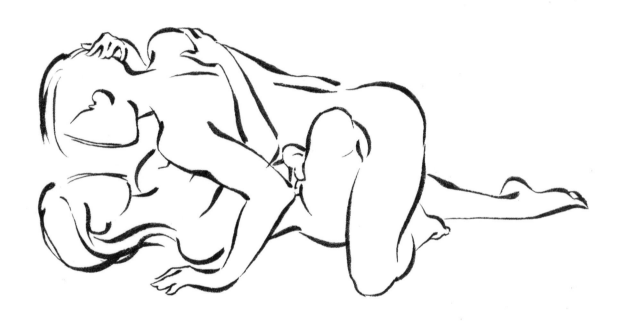

6.7 THE **ROWING BOAT**

Another upright sitting variation where both are face to face is the Rowing Boat. The couple will get out of the actual cross-legged position but are still sitting down, facing one another. Depending on the angle and size of his penis, it might be easier if he starts lying down. She can then straddle him to get his penis inside her. Once inside, she can slide down below his pelvis, so she is sitting on the floor, and simultaneously he will rise to sit. While upright, his legs will be outside her hips, and her legs will be over his thighs.

what she can do: For more support, she can slide her arms under his knees and grab on to her thighs. She can also wrap her legs around him and lean back on her hands for support.

what he can do: His arms can slip under her calves and knees. He can also use his hands under her bottom to guide the thrusting. However, not all penis shapes and sizes will take to this variation. His penis may slip out. If it is even slightly painful he should not attempt this.

BONUS!

Half the fun may be trying to get into and stay in this position. Sex is generally a combination of pleasurable feelings mixed with moments of awkwardness. Awkwardness tends to dissipate the more aroused the partners are, and laughter is also great for building intimacy between couples.

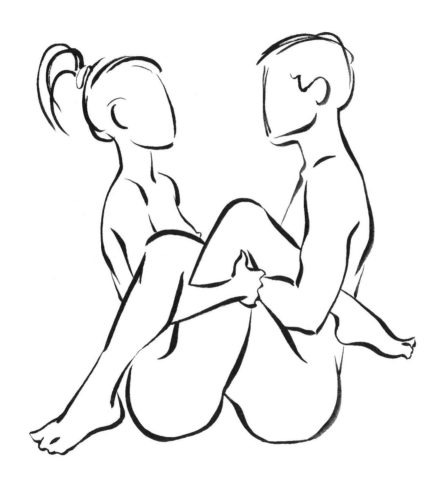

(6.8) THE **STAR**

If the Rowing Boat is too difficult, try this variation instead, an easy position to get into from the Rowing Boat. She just lies back and stretches one leg out, keeping the other bent. He can lower his knees so they are resting on the bed. He lifts her stretched-out leg under the hip and elevates her toward him with his thigh. He leans back on his hands for support.

what she can do: She can let him do the work in this position, and because her hands are free, she can focus on her own nipples, or reach up to touch his nipples. She is also free to stimulate her clitoris with her hands or with a vibrator. She might also just lie back, using her hands as a pillow, and enjoy the ride.

what he can do: He can watch her facial expressions as he goes in and out of her, and opt for slow, deep thrusts combined with some short and shallow thrusts to tease and arouse her. When she is ready he can speed up and completely lose control. All the visuals in this position should be highly arousing for him.

> **BONUS!**
>
> Turn up the kink! He can pull his penis out of her and while holding it, rub the tip/head against her clitoris, starting light and slow to tease and then getting harder and faster as she gets more and more excited.

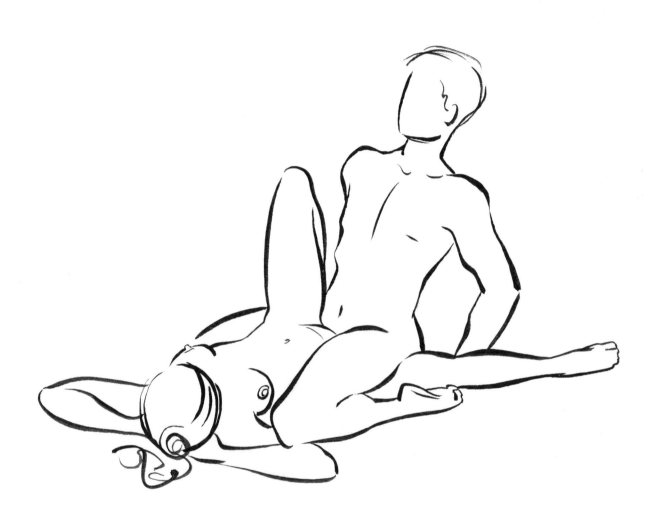

6.9 THE **TRIUMPH ARCH**

This position requires a bit of flexibility on both their parts. The man sits with his legs outstretched in front of him. The woman straddles him while on her knees. He penetrates her while she is still upright and then she leans backward until she is lying down. He then leans forward over her torso. There is still a lot of intimacy in this position and a lot of skin-to-skin contact.

what she can do: If her bent knees become painful or uncomfortable, she can straighten her legs out or place her feet on the bed with her knees pointing up.

what he can do: He is in the perfect position to nuzzle and kiss her breasts. He can place his hands beneath her back and pull her up toward him or use his body weight to hold her down and move inside her. Depending on the size and length of his penis, this angle could be excellent for G-spot stimulation.

> **BONUS!**
>
> He is in complete control as he guides her body onto his penis. This position should be called the *damsel in distress* because she really has the ability to surrender and let him take charge. She is at his mercy here, so he can use his strength to engage in his slowest grind.

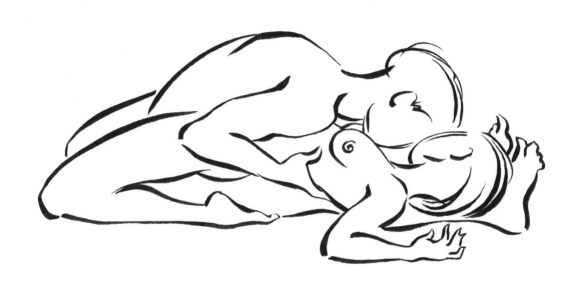

(6.10) THE **ROCKING HORSE**

In this variation, he sits cross-legged and leans back on his arms for support. She straddles him from a kneeling position and then sits down on his lap. From here, she rocks back and forth.

what she can do: She can place her hands on his shoulders to help her control the thrusting and bounce herself up and down on his penis. She sets the tone, speed, motion, and depth of thrusting. Deep kissing is a great way to build and maintain heat. Because their faces are close together she can initiate a make-out session.

what he can do: Using his hands as support he can help out by rocking back and forth. He can take a break and let her take charge. Because his hands are supporting him, they are essentially tied. To free up his hands he can lean against a wall. Once his hands are free he can return favors in most any way he chooses.

> ### BONUS!
>
> She is in a great position to pleasure him orally. She can slide back on her knees a bit so she can kiss and lick his neck, chest, stomach, and thighs and then take his penis in her mouth while she gently caresses his testicles.

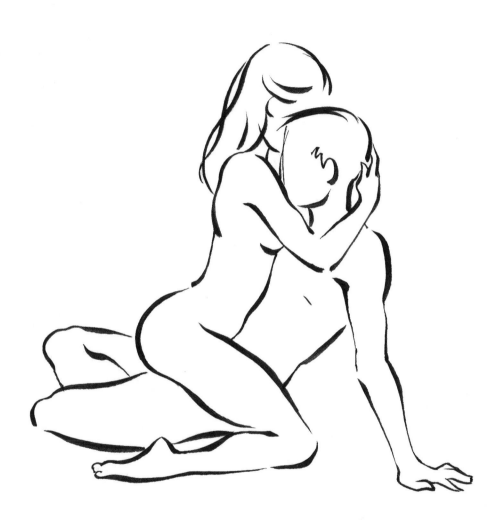

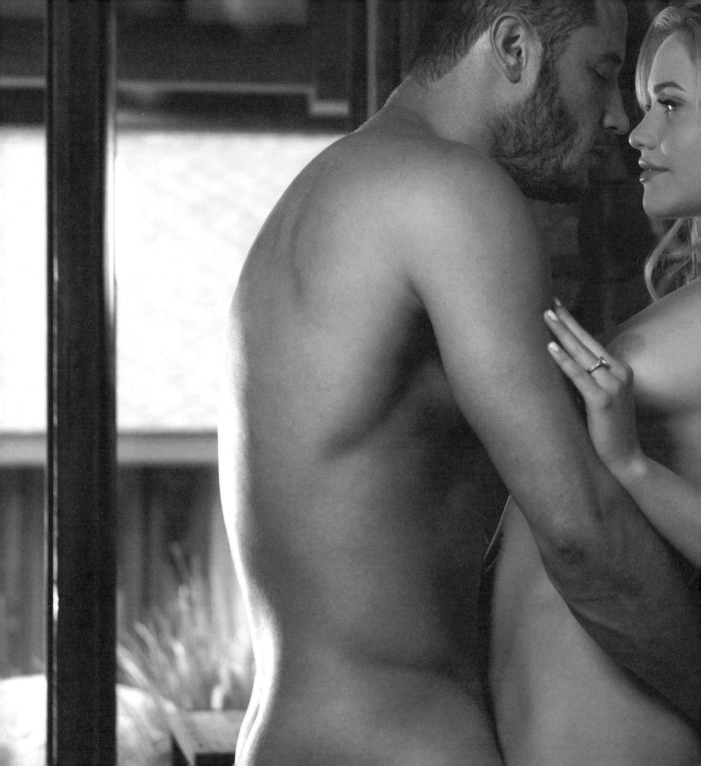

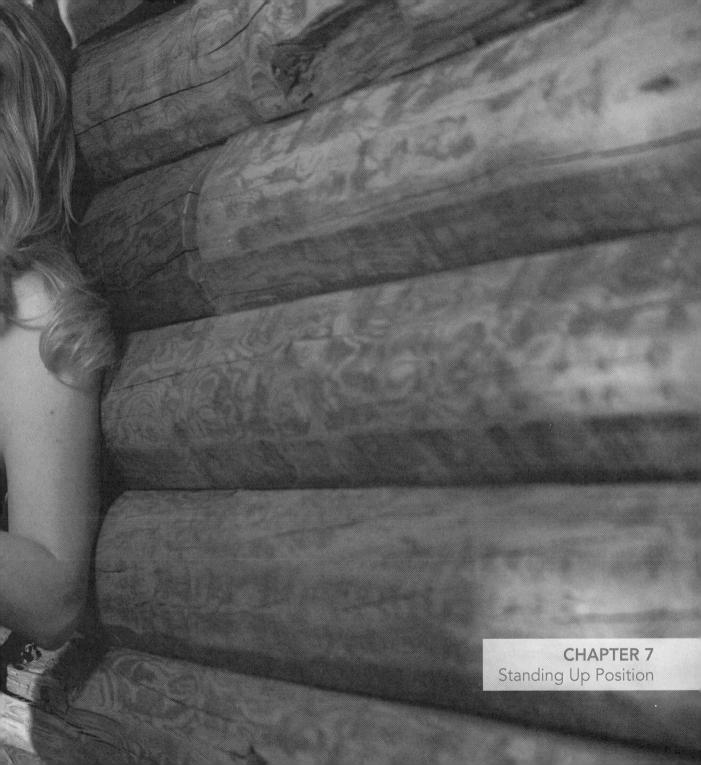

STANDING UP POSITION

HAVING SEX STANDING UP conjures the idea of spontaneity and unbridled passion. It might happen in the kitchen, in the shower, or maybe as a quickie in the elevator or a dark alleyway (like in the movie *9½ Weeks*). For exhibitionists, standing-up sex might occur on the balcony of their apartment or in the back hallway of a bar. Hollywood movies especially like to portray this position, hyping up a correlation between romance and spontaneous sex.

In actuality, this may be more fantasy than reality. Standing-up sex is great for daring and adventurous lovers, but the one thing that is missing from many of these upright positions is the aspect of stability, which comes from a bed or flat surface. And because many upright positions require some strength, engaging in one of these positions may be more difficult than what is portrayed in the movies.

Standing positions often happen in the heat of the moment; there is an element of surprise, along with the thrill of potentially getting caught if the couple is somewhere public. Better to mimic the idea of "dangerous" sex in an otherwise safe environment, such as your own home. Face-to-face standing sex is great for intimacy and kissing. In fact, this position may actually get started because a couple has a make-out session and takes it to the next level. This position has all the makings for steamy, hot, passionate, and lusty sex.

How to Do It

Both partners stand face to face. It might be helpful if she is standing with her back against a wall. She stands with her legs apart. He stands between her legs, lifts one of her legs, and enters her. The more aroused she is, the easier this position will be. She can bend her knee and put her foot behind her on the wall to get more support and traction while he thrusts. If she is strong enough, she can lift both feet and place them on the wall behind her. Finding something to hold on to, such as a doorknob, a railing, or a piece of furniture, can help as well. A square or narrow shower with two walls is great. She can lean her back on one and prop her feet up on the other. A doorway is also great for similar reasons. A narrow hallway or narrow kitchen might work as well.

Height might be an issue. The closer the two are in height, the easier standing positions will be. However, if the couple can't find a good fit, or something to hold on to, then there is a chance of the penis slipping out. Unless he is holding her up or supporting her in some way she will have to find a way to support herself, which may require some strength on her part.

benefits for her
Because this position can seem passionate and spontaneous, she may feel a sense of abandoning her inhibitions and really letting go.

benefits for him
Men who are able to maintain this position may enjoy an increased sense of confidence and prowess. Thrusting and holding this position at the same time may prove to be somewhat difficult, which makes this position all the more exciting for thrill-seekers and those looking for a challenge.

A BIT OF HISTORY

The Standing Up sex position can be easily traced back to ancient Indian culture, where having sex while standing up was seen as highly erotic and sensual. The erotic statues in ancient India's ruins and temples depict the beauty and grace of many of the variations of this position. In the Kama Sutra, a text that also originated in ancient India, sex standing up was considered a position reserved for only gods and deities and those who were closest to reaching nirvana. Because of its difficult nature and salacious and seductive properties, it was seen as somewhat taboo and only meant for the most sexually aware and open.

7.1 **STANDING UP, MAN BEHIND**

In this variation the man stands behind her with his knees slightly bent. She faces a wall in front of her and can place her hands on the wall for stability. She spreads her legs, he moves between her legs, and enters her from there.

what she can do: She can lean her pelvis back into him to get the perfect angle, or move forward and arch her back if that feels better. This is a great time to feel the pleasure of being "taken."

what he can do: This position can hit her G-spot, so he can pull back his thrusts, make them shorter if it feels good to her, or make them deeper if that is what she wants. He can also do a combination of the two, and speed up when he needs a faster thrust. With her back to him, and her legs spread, he can use his fingers to stimulate her before intercourse or during a break to build excitement. He can take his penis out, use his fingers for a bit, and then reenter her.

> **BONUS!**
>
> This position might be sexiest if it happens spontaneously, such as right when a partner walks in the door. He can grab her, tell her something dirty (or sexy or romantic), and then either tell her to put her hands against the wall or help her out with it. Feel the rush of sexual energy.

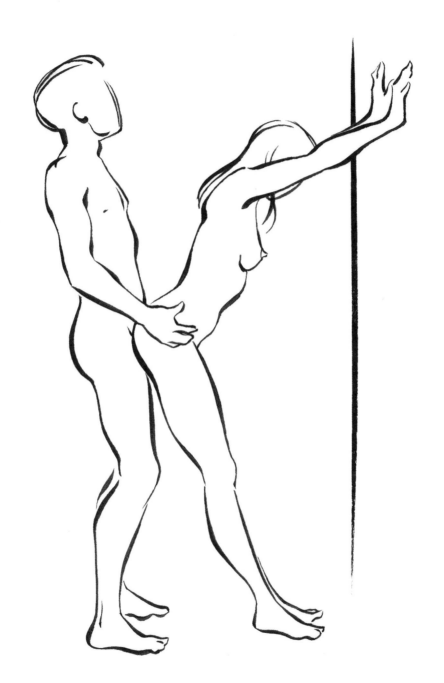

7.2 STANDING **DOGGY**

In Standing Doggy, she hinges over at the waist and uses a chair, sofa, table, or bed to support her arms. He grabs her from the waist and enters her from behind.

what she can do: She can control the angle by arching her back, rounding her back, or lengthening her arms out in front of her. She can also encourage a different kind of thrust by circling her hips or alternating circles with back-and-forth thrusts.

what he can do: As with many of the Doggy-Style and rear-entry positions, this position doesn't hit many of her erogenous spots. Thus he can slow his movements and use shallow thrusts combined with deeper thrusts to give her G-spot a little massage. He can reach over and stimulate her clitoris or nipples.

> **BONUS!**
>
> Has she been naughty? She might need to be bent over a chair or sofa and shown some discipline. If she is wearing a skirt with no panties, she will be ready to get what she deserves.

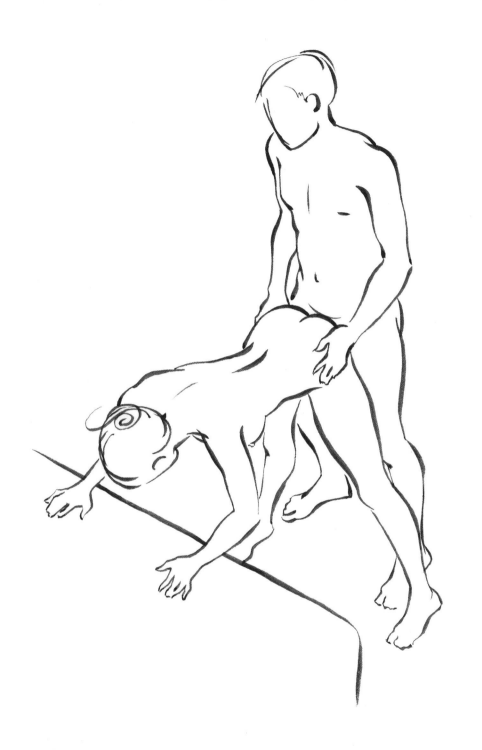

(7.3) LADY **LEG LIFT**

This challenging standing variation may seem more like an acrobatic pose than a sex position. Again, this position will be easier if there is a wall for one of them to lean against for support. Doing this without some form of support may prove difficult for some and quite impossible for many. The partners stand face to face with his legs about shoulder width apart and his knees slightly bent. She wraps her arms around his neck and raises one leg up onto his shoulder. He holds her hips or her back and enters her from there.

what she can do: She will need to be pretty flexible to do the leg lift. If she can't get her leg up onto his shoulder, she can place her foot against the wall instead.

what he can do: If she is super flexible, this will be a fun position for him. He will have good access to her G-spot and will be able to glide in with a direct thrust. He can lean back against a wall, which will give her a lot more control and stability.

> **BONUS!**
>
> As with all standing positions, the couple's relative heights will make a big difference in whether this is successful. One option is to have the taller person stand at the base of the stairs and the shorter person move up a step. The banister and the wall can provide needed support.

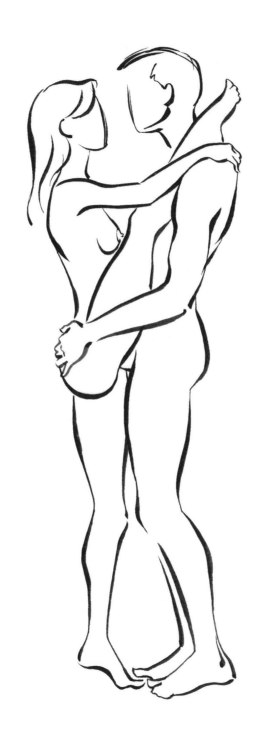

THE PADLOCK

The Padlock variation is a definite go-to position of Hollywood movies but is also an easy, fun, and spontaneous one that can be done at home in practically any room. She finds a surface to sit on, such as a kitchen or bathroom counter, a table, or a washing machine, and pushes herself up onto it (or he can lift her up and place her there). He approaches between her legs and enters her. The height should be easy enough for him to access her directly. Both can gaze into each other's eyes to intensify the moment. Because this does not take place in a bed, and perhaps not even in the bedroom, this has the essence of forbidden sex, which can make this position exciting.

what she can do: She can lean back on her hands to support herself and wrap her legs around him to make it easier to ride the motion.

what he can do: He can grab her hips and pull her closer to him. If the surface is low and he is too tall, he can take a step backward and lean into her to lower his pelvis.

BONUS!

Couples can role-play to bring excitement back into the bedroom, and this position is one that is prime for a little fantasy. What illicit or taboo fantasy does this position bring to mind? Create a story and build on it. Or, keep it simple and start with her clothes on and frantically take them off her while getting into this position. If she's on the washer or dryer, try this when the machine is running for some extra heat and vibration.

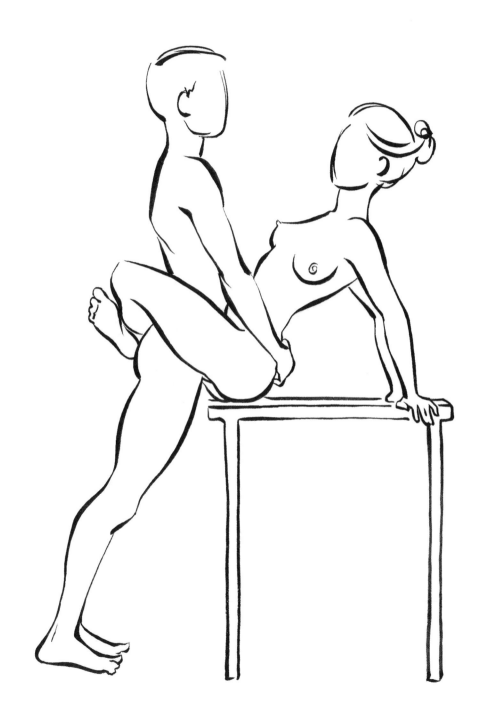

(7.5) CARTING

For men who enjoy working out and weightlifting, this position provides the opportunity to show off those muscles. Carting requires a lot of strength and stamina, and is probably not going to work for everyone. There are a few ways to get into this position. The two can stand face to face as he lifts her up one leg at a time. She may also be carried from a seated position. The couple will ultimately end up in a position where he is carrying her. He can support her under her bottom, and she can wrap her legs around his waist and her arms around his neck. This is a great way for him to carry her from one sexy location to the next.

what she can do: Feeling his masculine power, she can step into her own feminine energy.

what he can do: If he is strong, this is a nice way for him to show off his muscles and step into his masculine energy.

BONUS!

This position requires a lot of strength and stamina and therefore will not work for everyone. If he can get her back against the wall, this position will be easier. The wall also adds a flavor of control, which can make this position even more enjoyable for both, increasing the power dynamic in his favor. Another thing to remember is adrenaline gives us strength. If the couple is having a heated moment, anything is possible.

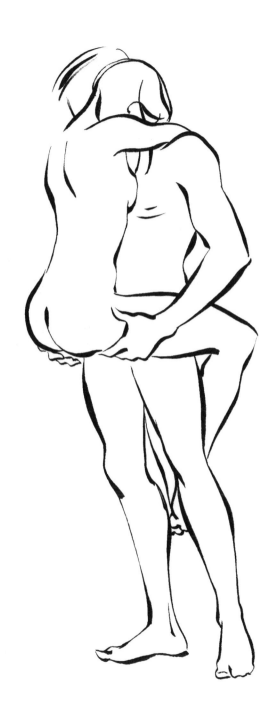

7.6 SUSPENDED **SCISSORS**

Another standing sex position that requires a lot of strength is a variation called Suspended Scissors. She lies on her side and scoots herself off the edge of the bed until her hand reaches the floor, with just her legs still on the bed. She supports herself with one arm and he holds her up from her waist. He steps behind her and, holding one of her legs up, enters her. Yes, this will happen while she is supporting herself on one arm. It does require a little extra body strength from both partners. Don't attempt this position if you're not feeling comfortable about it, as thrusting and penetration while holding a standing position can sometimes feel like a Herculean feat.

what she can do: If he is steady, she can use her other arm to hold onto him. She will need some adrenaline to get into and stay in this position, and if she is turned on this can be a lot of fun. The angle of this position is also great for hitting her G-spot.

what he can do: He will have to assist in holding her up. He can hold on to her waist or mid-back from behind her or wrap one arm around her front while entering from the back. The bed will provide the rest of the support.

> **BONUS!**
>
> He is in a great position to play with her vulva and finger her clitoris.

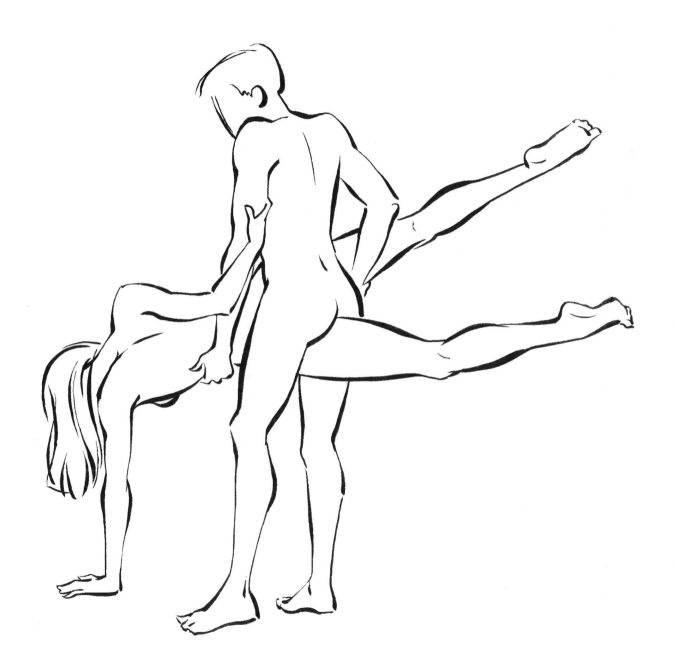

7.7 THE **INDIAN** HEADSTAND

This variation requires strength on his part and may be even more fun if she has good arm strength. She puts all her weight on her hands stretched out in front of her about shoulder-width apart, as though she is about to attempt a handstand. (She is really in more of a handstand than headstand for this position.) The man stands on the floor behind her. She can either kick her legs up and let him catch her and lift her by the hips or he can help her by guiding her hips into position. She then puts her legs under his arms and he enters her from there.

what she can do: It may seem that both partners need a lot of strength and flexibility for this position, but it also may be achieved if she relaxes her body and is able to trust him to hold her. Adrenaline, arousal, and the heat of the moment can make this position a little easier to manage.

what he can do: If he is strong enough he will love the control and energy this pose inspires, not to mention the great views of her backside.

> ### BONUS!
>
> Because there is little in terms of eye contact and both partners' hands are occupied, stimulating other erotic zones will not be possible. This is where dirty talk can make all the difference. He can tell her what he is doing to her and she can tell him how it feels or what she wants. This will heighten arousal and communication even though they can't see each other's faces.

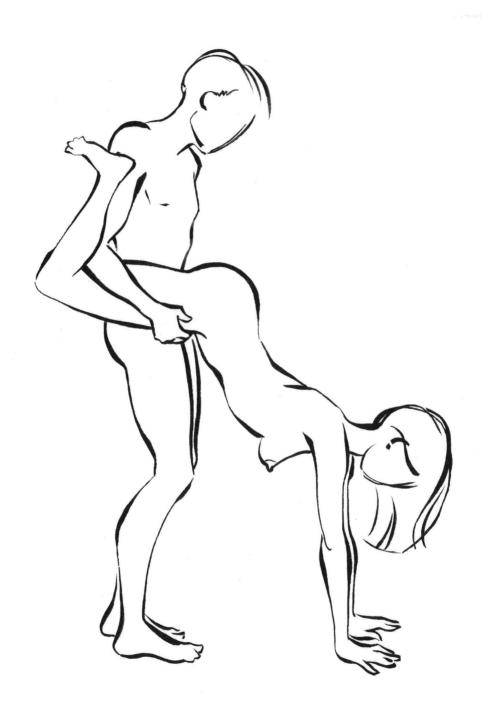

7.8 THE **SQUAT BALANCE**

This is a standing sex position that requires some skill and strength but can be really exciting if he loves to grab her ass and she loves having her butt massaged and squeezed during sex. The woman stands on the bed, a table, or a chair (facing the back of the chair) with her back to the man. He stands behind her and places his hands under her bottom for support. She squats down onto him, leans back against his chest, and holds onto him with her arms. He supports her body and penetrates her at the same time.

what she can do: She can tilt her pelvis forward to hit her G-spot. Since the bed and his arms are her only supports, her legs could get tired in this position, even if she is strong.

what he can do: Men like having a woman squat on their penis. He can control her motions and has a great view of sliding in and out of her vagina. If he leans forward and looks over her shoulder, he will have a nice view of her vulva. He can also kiss her neck and shoulders to add some sensuality to this position. Even with good arm strength, it might become tiring for him to hold her up while maintaining a good position for intercourse.

> ### BONUS!
>
> For those who like ass play, this can be a fun position. He can squeeze and separate her cheeks, run his fingers along her crack, and stroke her anus. If she enjoys it, he might slip a finger inside her anus to add another level of sensation.

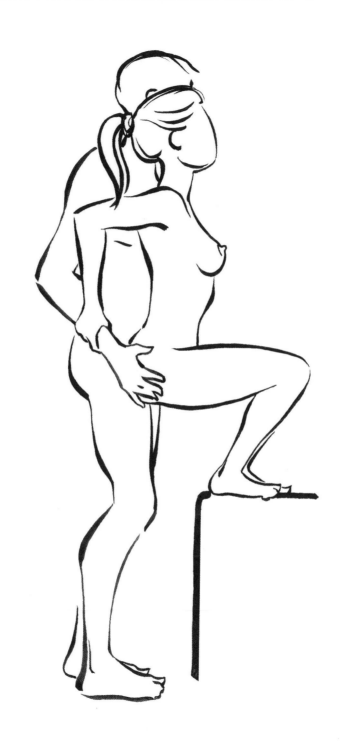

7.9 THE **VENUS NECKLACE**

In the Venus Necklace, she sits on a table, the edge of the bed, or a chair and leans back. She raises her legs up to his shoulders and wraps her ankles around the back of his neck. He can then enter her from this position.

what she can do: She can alter the angle of penetration by switching the position of her arms, such as propping herself up on her elbows or coming up onto her hands. If holding her weight on her arms gets tiring, she can lean on a pillow or they can move to a softer surface.

what he can do: This variation has the potential for vigorous and deep penetration, since he won't have to support her.

BONUS!

Going down on her is easy from this position. He can let her legs dangle over his shoulders while using his tongue on her clitoris and labia. This is a great way to take a break from the intensity of intercourse if he feels he may come too soon. If she likes it, he can insert two fingers in her vagina and stimulate her G-spot while tasting her with his tongue.

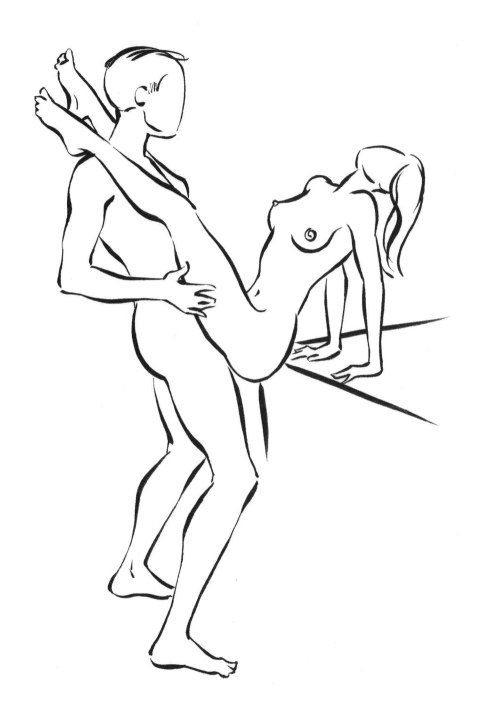

(7.10) THE FRISK

In this sexy standing-up pose, she stands with her hands against a wall, bending slightly forward, feet apart. He approaches her from behind as though he is going to frisk her. This position is perfect for tight spaces, like showers and hallways. It is also great for those in a rush. For an added thrill, try this right when you walk through the door or right before leaving.

what she can do: She can control the angle and depth of penetration by moving her hips toward him or away from him and arching her back, which may stimulate her G-spot.

what he can do: From behind he has control of his movements and his hands are free to wander her body. He can grab her hair and spank her lightly to add more intensity to this position.

BONUS!

The Frisk is like a body search, which might provide some ideas for fantasy and role-play. Perhaps he pulls her over on the highway and has reason to frisk her up against her car. Or perhaps she is being brought into the station and he is a corrupt cop who demands a little favor before he'll let her go.

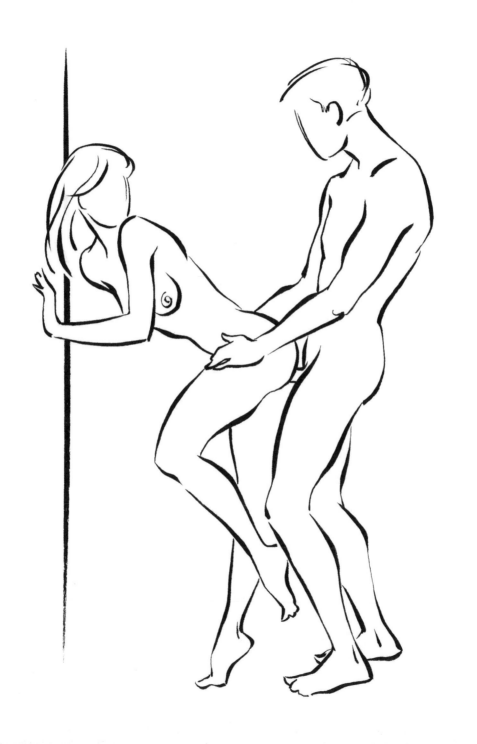

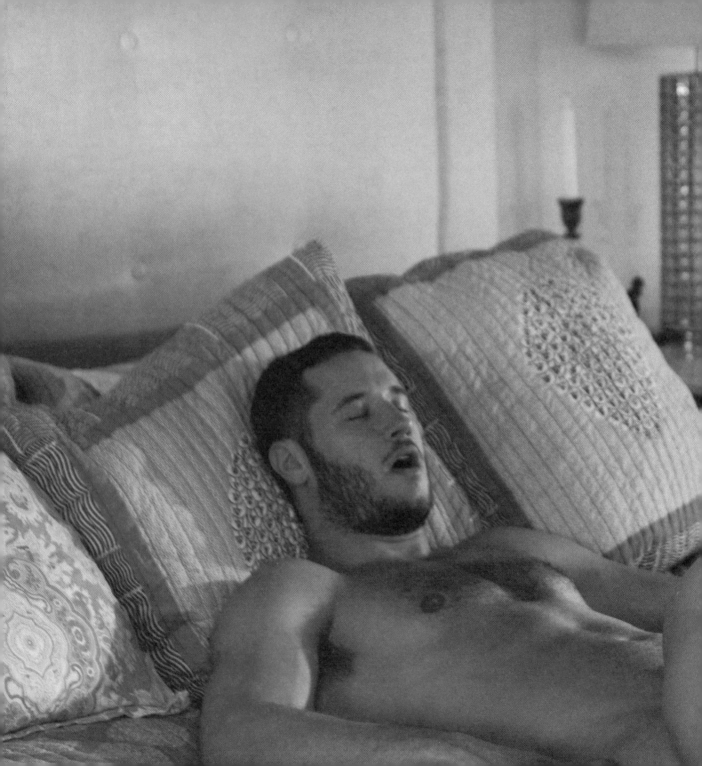

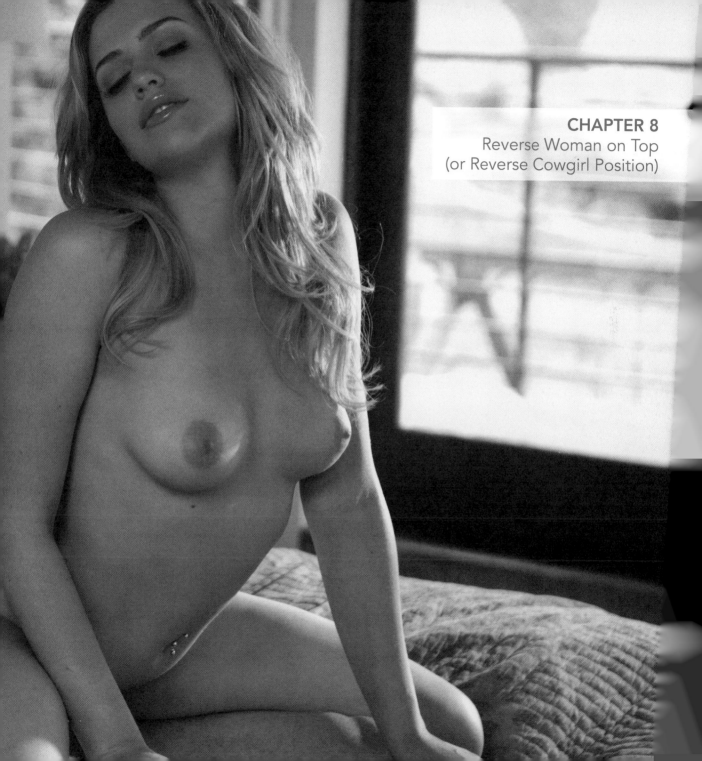

CHAPTER 8
Reverse Woman on Top
(or Reverse Cowgirl Position)

REVERSE WOMAN ON TOP
(OR REVERSE COWGIRL POSITION)

THIS SET OF SEX POSITIONS is built around the popular Reverse Cowgirl position. Woman-on-top positions are popular in today's culture because of the feminist qualities they embrace. When she is on top, she is in charge of her sexuality and her pleasure. Women are being encouraged to embrace their bodies as they are and to let their partners know what they like and want in the bedroom. Woman-on-top reminds us that she can enjoy sex just as much as any man.

Woman-on-top allows for role reversal. Men enjoy and appreciate being on the bottom and letting her take the reins, and women feel empowered in positions where they are in charge. Sometimes women shy away from woman-on-top positions if they feel less experienced, awkward, or shy about their bodies. Reverse Cowgirl will allow her to discover what feels good in a less intimate way, because she is facing away from him, and this position is perfect if she is feeling like she wants to be in her own head for a while.

How to Do It

He lies down on his back. He can prop himself up on some pillows or sit up. His legs are straight out in front of him. She straddles him, facing toward his feet. She can put her hands outside his legs to get some support. She can bend forward or lean back to find the right angle for G-spot stimulation and to hit other sensitive areas.

benefits for her

In this position, she gets to control the speed and depth of penetration. If she is not using her hands to move up and down, she can also stimulate herself in this position. Moving to her feet in this position, while still staying on his penis, gives way to the squat.

benefits for him

Men tend to love this position just as much as women do. He gets to watch her ass and her entire body moving up and down on his penis. This is arousing in itself. If he happens to be sitting up, he can use his hands to stimulate her breasts or nipples. He can also reach down and stimulate her clitoris with his hands or use a vibrator. By holding her hips, he can guide her in a rhythm and speed that feel good to him, and he can try making circles with his own hips to hit her various erogenous zones.

A BIT OF HISTORY

The Reverse Woman-on-Top position has been around for a long time, and depictions of this position have been found in ancient Egyptian and Indian art. Woman on Top as a position was deemed evil and outside the realm of acceptable sexual practices for procreation, punishable by three years of penance in Medieval Judeo-Christian history, in England, Ireland, and France. Meanwhile, Reverse Woman on Top was deemed the most "deviant" of all, sometimes punishable by death. It is interesting to note that while many sex acts, including Reverse Woman-on-Top position, adultery, and homosexuality, were illegal, prostitution was often legal, and poems and art often depicted these more deviant sexual acts quite succinctly. The message was definitely "look, but don't touch." If these otherwise non-permissible acts, such as the Reverse Woman on Top, took place outside of wedlock, marriage itself was considered penance.

8.1 THE **BREASTSTROKE**

In this variation, he remains lying down. He can have a pillow under his head for support. She lies face down on him, facing his feet. The position is called the breaststroke because she can move her legs like she is swimming to engage her pelvic muscles. As she opens and closes her legs, the muscles around her vagina naturally expand and contract, stimulating both partners.

what they can do: Try this position in the pool. Instead of him lying on his back, he can stand in the shallow end of the pool so his penis is just below the water. He can hold on to her waist. She then spreads her legs to do the open and closing motion of the breaststroke. Maybe it was meant for this!

> ### BONUS!
>
> The angle in this position is excellent for hitting her G-spot. Some women say that having pressure on their G-spot makes it feel like they are going to urinate. The G-spot is located near the urethral glands, a little bit above the pelvic bone, and so this sensation is quite common. Typically, the feeling will pass. If it does not, feel free to go relieve yourself. Remember to relax. Some women have intense orgasms from G-spot stimulation, and some women don't like the intensity at all. And some women do ejaculate from G-spot stimulation. This is also quite normal, and the ejaculate should not be confused with urine.

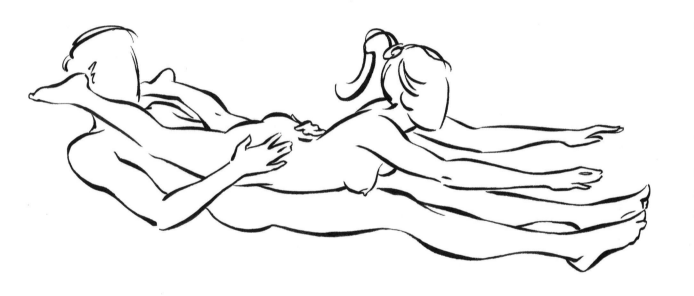

THE PRONE TIGER

This is a nice variation of the Reverse Woman on Top. The man sits on the bed with his legs outstretched. She straddles his body, her back to him. She lowers herself down onto his penis, then leans forward so her torso is lying on his legs or between his legs. She then stretches her legs out as straight as possible. This is another great G-spot stimulator.

what she can do: She can wrap her arms around his legs or grab his feet for leverage and stability. She can rock back and forth on his penis, lift herself up on her hands to alter the angle, or lift up her hips and move them in a circular motion or figure eight.

what he can do: He is face to face with her bottom. He can caress her ass or even spank it lightly to add some gusto to the position. He may also lean back on his forearms and elbows to simply enjoy the view.

> **BONUS!**
>
> Getting intimate when her face is down near his feet may seem challenging, but there are ways to make this position sensual. Because she is near his feet, this is a good opportunity for her to caress, lick, and kiss them. The feet have a lot of nerve endings, and light kisses can feel tantalizing, building tension and arousal.

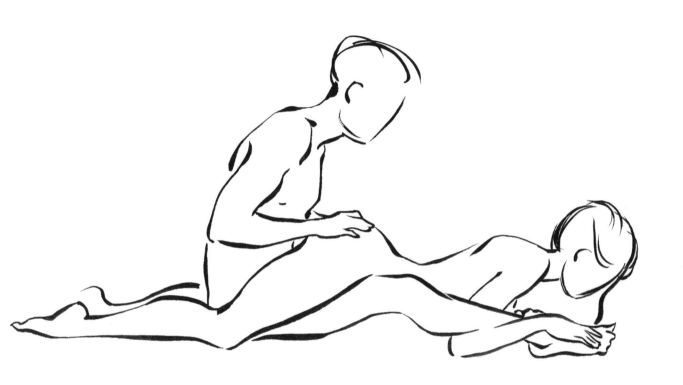

(8.3) THE GALLEY

In this variation of the Reverse Woman on Top, he sits with his legs forward and leans back on his arms. She lies down on his legs, straddling him at the hips. It is similar to the Prone Tiger, but in this position she unwraps her arms and uses them as support. Her legs will stretch back out, but they can be bent at the knees for more support. The extra support in this position gives her a lot more stability to guide the thrusting and maneuver her hips.

what she can do: Women who like a little bit of bottom action will enjoy this, as it places her butt close to his face, making it easy for him to lick and caress her ass all over.

what he can do: Watching her on all fours moving back and forth on his penis can be a thrill. Men love watching a woman who is enjoying herself sexually, and she is fully in charge in this position. He can place his hands on her bum and push her back and forth to change things up a bit.

BONUS!

Men who enjoy a little bit of anal play can get into this position, inserting a finger into her anus during intercourse and licking and kissing her butt cheeks. There are plenty of anal toys to be enjoyed, too, such as butt plugs, anal beads, and dildos. There are also anal starter kits for those who are new to backdoor play; start with the smallest butt plug in the kit (there are usually three: small, medium, and large) and work your way up in size as you get more comfortable.

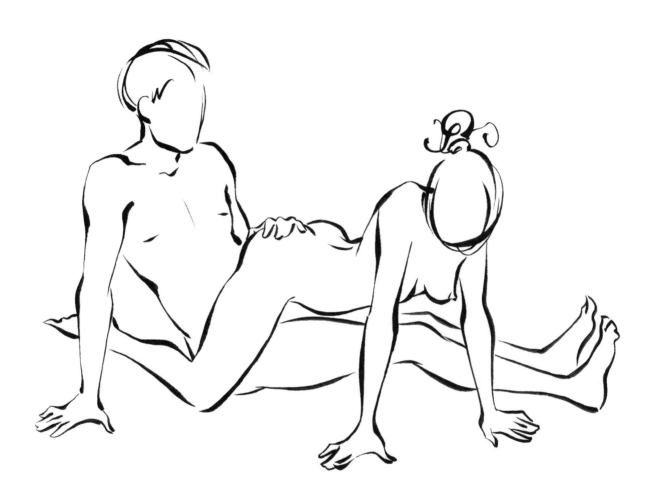

8.4 THE **RIDER**

This variation is slightly different from Reverse Cowgirl and gives her more access to his pleasure zones. He lies on his back and may use a pillow to support his head. She straddles him and places her knees on either side of him. Instead of being upright (as in Reverse Cowgirl), she leans forward to balance herself on his knees. He holds her hips as they move together.

what she can do: Her hands are free, so she can reach over to play with his scrotum and lightly handle his testicles. She can also stroke his perineum (the area between his testicles and his anus).

what he can do: He can worship the beautiful butt that is right in front of him, sliding his fingers along her crack and fingering the entrance to her anus.

BONUS!

When it comes to certain types of sex play, particularly in areas the couple has not explored or discussed but that are introduced in the midst of intimacy, it is important to rely on nonverbal communication, such as body language and sounds. This is even more true when the partners are not facing each other, as in this position. It is always best to be gentle, go slow, and wait for cues. Once you get the green light, such as "oh, yes" or moans of pleasure, you know you can continue. Any signs of discomfort, such as moving away from the stimulation, indicate that it's time to stop and check in. A simple "Does this feel good?" or "Do you like this?" can get the conversation started.

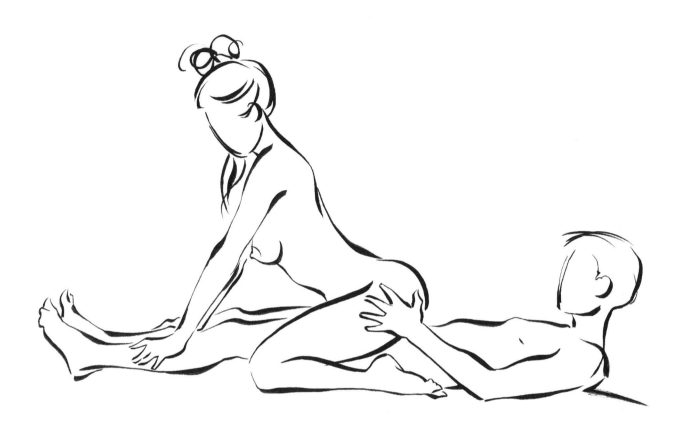

8.5 THE SEATED **WHEELBARROW**

This position has the potential to be a sexy yet animalistic variation of Reverse Woman on Top, with a twist. He sits on the edge of the bed or a chair. She can start out straddling him and sitting on his lap, with her back to him. From here, he can hold on to her hips. Penetration can even start here, but eventually she tilts her body downward until her hands reach the floor and her arms support her in a sort of table position. Her legs remain on the bed. He lifts her up by her pelvis so she can wrap her legs around his waist.

what she can do: She can gyrate her hips in a circular motion or move her torso forward and back. This angle has the potential to go deep, hitting her A-spot on the anterior wall of the vagina.

what he can do: He has excellent views from here. He can enjoy watching her body and head move back and forth. He should provide stability by holding her waist, and making sure her thighs are resting firmly on his.

> **BONUS!**
>
> If she feels safe and comfortable with him, both physically and emotionally, she can let herself lose control in this position. He can encourage her by reminding her how sexy she looks, not just in the moment but at other times as well. She can move her head and neck around to let her animalistic side out and thus give him the show of a lifetime. The end result when two people share extreme pleasure based on trust, respect, and mutual admiration can lead to an intense, intimate bond.

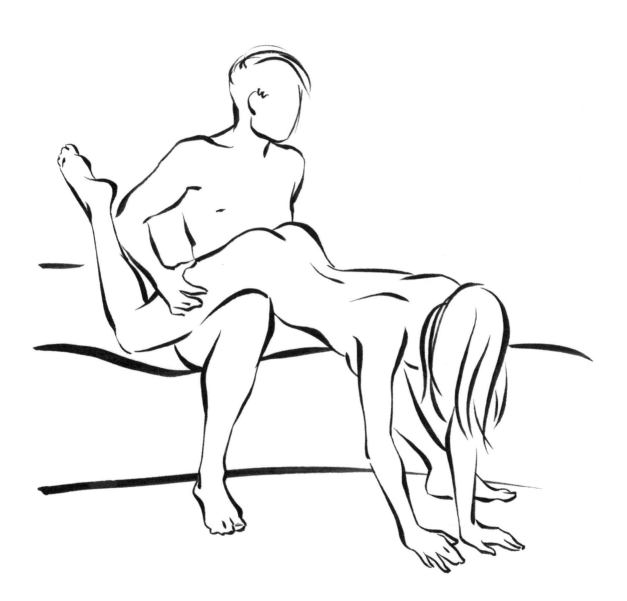

8.6 THE STANDING **WHEELBARROW**

The previous position, the Seated Wheelbarrow, is a good starting point for this variation, the standing wheelbarrow. The couple can get into this position if he simply moves from a seated to a standing position and carefully brings her with him. When she is steady, she can wrap her legs around his waist. Or, to get into this position if he is already standing, she gets onto all fours and he enters her as if he were in standing doggy or rear entry. Then, when she is ready, he lifts her up by the hips, steadies her, and she wraps her legs around his waist. This position can also be done with him holding her feet while her legs are bent, as though he were pushing a wheelbarrow.

what she can do: Because his hands are holding on to her and her hands are trying to balance in this position, there is not a lot of room for extra stimulation. She can exercise her pubococcygeus (PC) muscles (her pelvic floor) by doing Kegel exercises—flexing and contracting her PC muscles—to give both of them more sensation. These exercises performed during sex can often help start an orgasm.

what he can do: It's important for him to use his strength and balance to bring stability to this position. If he feels his energy flagging, he can sit down on the edge of the bed or a chair or very gently lower her to the floor.

> ### BONUS!
>
> Strengthening the PC muscles can help men and women gain more control during sex. To do this, start out by locating this muscle, which lies along the pelvic floor. While urinating, or when you have the urge to pee, squeeze the muscle, which stops the flow of urine. Other muscles should be relaxed, such as the stomach and leg muscles. Then breathe in and out while contracting and releasing the PC muscle to encourage greater control of your sexual stamina for men, and degree of orgasm for women.

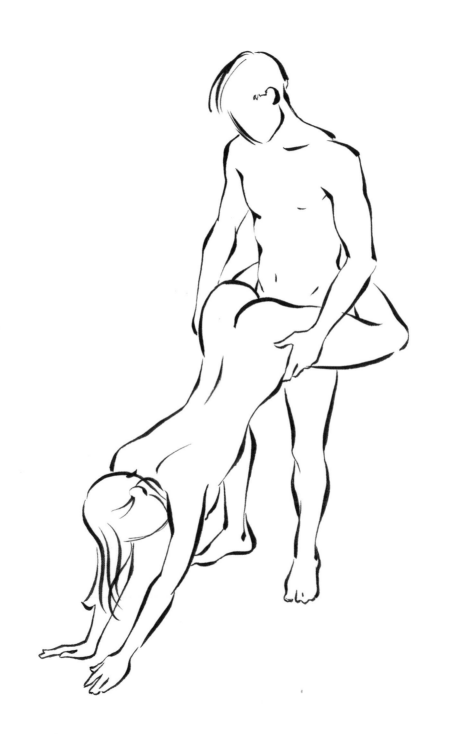

8.7 THE COUCH SURFER

This position requires a couch or sofa, so find a comfortable one with a good armrest. She bends herself over the armrest. He positions himself behind her. Once he penetrates her, she puts her legs between his. Crossing her legs at the ankles tightens her vaginal entrance, which will make for a snugger sensation.

what she can do: She has a lot of nearby cushions to provide support and comfort for her head. She can also grab on to the cushions with her hands and grind herself against the armrest. She will love the varieties of penetration—shallow for G-spot stimulation or deeper for A-spot stimulation; both are likely scenarios in this position.

what he can do: He needs to be mindful of the angle and the force of his thrusting to make sure the position is not hurting her back or neck. He will love the view of her bottom.

> **BONUS!**
>
> As a standing sex position, the couch surfer has the added benefit of being perfect for a quickie in the middle of the day or right before heading off to work in the morning.

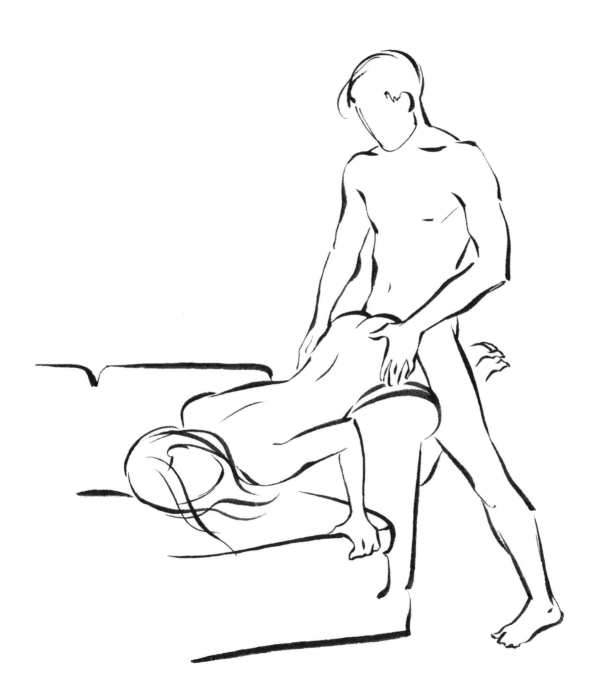

8.8 SEATED OR **REVERSE** WOMAN-ON-TOP SCISSORS

This is similar to Reverse Cowgirl, with a slight variation. To get into position, he lies on his back with his knees bent. He can use a pillow under his head for support. She straddles him, facing his feet, with one leg between his legs and the other leg on the outside of his hip. She may use his knee as support.

what she can do: She has control of the depth, speed, and motion in this position. She can move up and down or in a circular motion and find an angle that hits her G-spot. His thigh between her legs provides the perfect spot to grind against and stimulate her clitoris. This position is excellent for simultaneous clitoral and G-spot orgasm.

what he can do: He will get to relax and enjoy the ride, if that is what he wants. Or he may opt for a more active approach where he participates in guiding the motion. He can prop himself up on his arms and reach around to stimulate her breasts, nipples, and clitoris. He is also in a great position to stimulate her anus with his finger.

> **BONUS!**
>
> She can tease him in this position by sitting only on the tip of his penis and then pulling herself up off his penis. She can look back over her shoulder at him to intensify her sense of power.

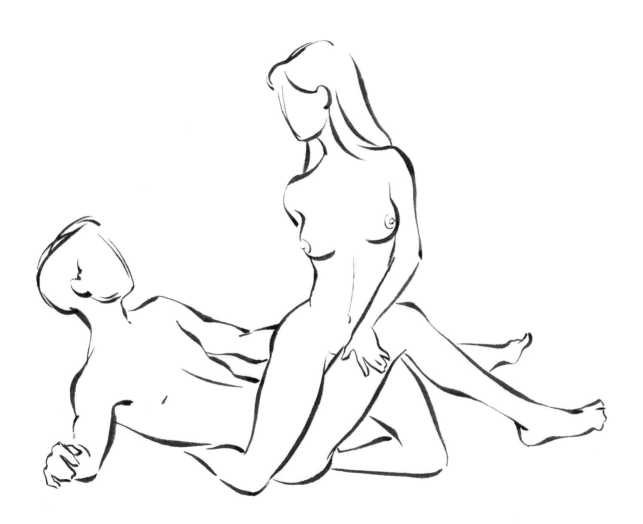

SNOW **ANGEL**

This upside-down version of Reverse Cowgirl is known as the Snow Angel. For a challenge, the couple can just roll over from the breaststroke position, so that she is now on the bottom and he is face down. If that is too difficult, she can lie on her back with her legs out straight. He straddles her, facing away, toward her feet. She wraps her legs around his back and tilts her pelvis up to allow for penetration.

what she can do: She gets a nice view of his butt in this position. She also has the benefit of seeing what is going on, whereas his vision is impaired from this angle. She can grab on to his ass to help him glide in and out of her—and to keep him inside her, as slipping out may happen in this position.

what he can do: This is not an easy position to maintain penetration, so he needs to be careful and make sure his penis does not slip out. If it does, he can just relax and let her engage in some anal play before moving into another position.

BONUS!

With his butt so close to her face and her hands free, it's her turn to engage in some anal play. She can grab and spank his bottom or lightly caress his testicles, perineum, and anus with her fingers. There are plenty of anal sex toys for him as well, some that target his P-spot (the prostate gland, located 1½ inches (3.8 cm) inside his anus toward the base of his penis), which she can also reach with her fingers. Massaging this walnut-size gland can give him a powerful orgasm.

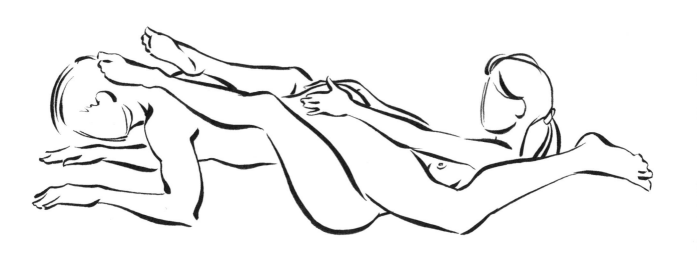

8.10 THE **TRANSATLANTIC**

This variation, at first glance, may look harder than it really is. If the partners have a little bit of body strength, this position can be pulled off and can provide some intense thrusting. He sits in a chair or on the edge of the bed or couch with his legs straight down (not bent at the knees). He pushes his hips out to make his bottom half as straight as possible. She lies on his lap with her back resting on his thighs. Her torso and chest will be parallel with his shins and lower legs. Her hands can be above her head on the floor, or she can place them on the chair for support. She wraps her legs around his neck. He may use his hands behind him for support.

what she can do: Despite lying down with her head almost touching the ground, she actually has quite a bit of control in this position. Her arms support her upper body, and she can use them to push her body up and down toward him. Her legs, which are resting on his shoulders, can also guide her body up toward him. The right angle could stimulate her G-spot.

what he can do: He can use his arms to push his pelvis toward her and aid in the thrusting.

> **BONUS!**
>
> If she is a fan of or a pro at anal sex, she will love this position. Raising her hips a little higher will give him direct access to her ass. He can move his penis gently inside of her and if she has the upper body strength, she can control some of the motion.

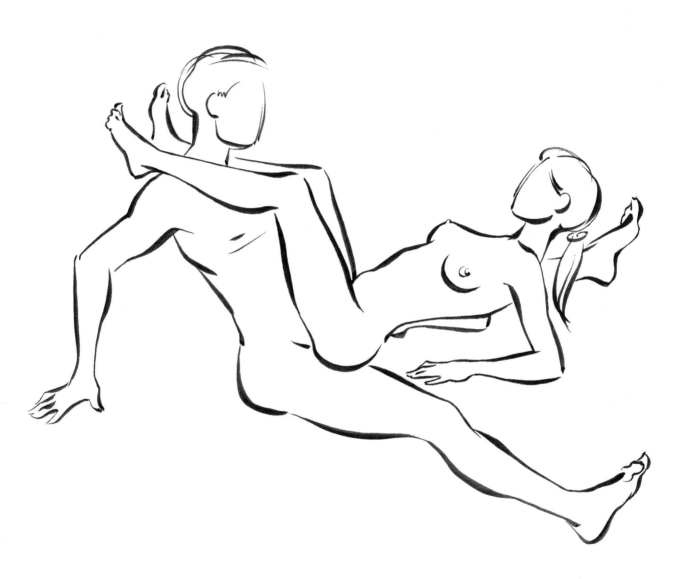

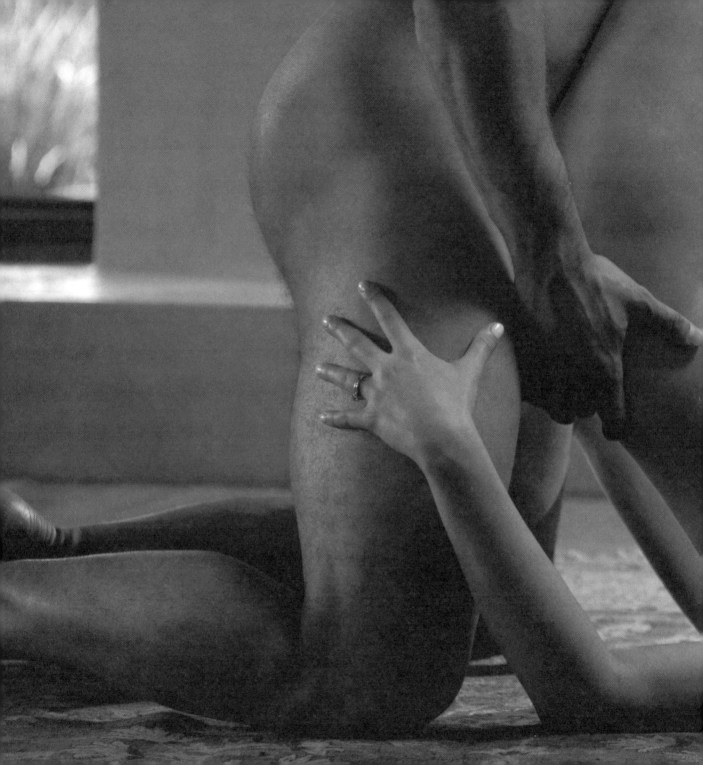

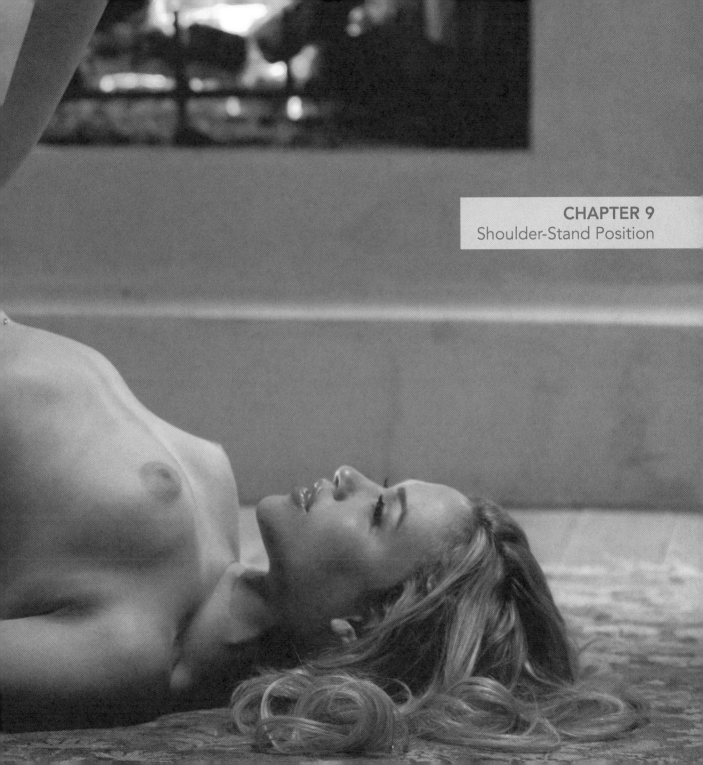

09

SHOULDER-STAND POSITION

SHOULDER-STAND SEX POSITIONS feature the woman in some form of a shoulder stand. Because she is on her shoulders, many of these poses have a similar foundation as Missionary position, but with a little less support, and have the appearance of being more creative and adventurous. While some of the Shoulder-Stand variations may seem and look more difficult at first glance, many of them are actually fairly easy and comfortable, and they bring fun variety into the bedroom.

Shoulder stands are used in the meditative spiritual sexuality practice known as Tantra. Tantra originated from Vedic traditions of Hinduism and is believed to have roots in ancient Buddhism. The tenets of tantric sex are about letting go of the ego, merging with your partner on a spiritual level, and, in most cases, delaying intercourse and orgasm. The individual learns to become one with the universe and earth and to channel sexual energy into spiritual energy while engaging in provocative sexual postures.

Physically speaking, Shoulder-Stand positions are great for the brain, the muscles, and the organs. In day-to-day life we are always standing, walking, and sitting upright. Shoulder stands change the pull of gravity on the blood and draw it toward your head. Yogis believe this aids circulation and restores and strengthens the immune system, ultimately bringing the body back to homeostasis.

Note: Shoulder stands are contraindicated for women who are pregnant and those with high blood pressure.

How to Do It

She starts by lying on her back and he kneels in front her. She can wrap her legs around his waist or torso and then he lifts her up so he can enter her. He supports her with one arm under her lower back while she straightens her legs and back and puts the weight on his shoulders. Because he is holding much of her body weight, he may get tired, and the weight placed on her cervical spine may cause undue pain and risk of neck injury, particularly if not done properly. Don't hesitate to use pillows and blankets for support in any of the Shoulder-Stand positions. He can use a blanket under his knees for support.

benefits for her

By arching her back, she tilts her pelvis forward as well, which will hit her G-spot. This position is good for deep penetration and an amazing orgasm. This can also be a good muscle toner for both partners.

benefits for him

He is in control in many of these Shoulder-Stand positions, allowing him to step into his masculine power. This is also great for building and showing off his body strength. Since he is supporting both their body weights, he gets twice the workout. He can work his arm muscles by holding her body weight and he can build his leg muscles by supporting his own body weight.

A BIT OF HISTORY

Shoulder stands were part of ancient yoga practices in India and are known as the Queen or Mother of restorative yoga postures. Most yoga postures are considered meditative and restorative, bringing calmness, balance, serenity, and peace of mind.

(9.1) THE **SLINGSHOT**

This first variation is often referred to as the *shoulder holder*, and is slightly easier than the Shoulder Stand itself. She lies on her back and puts her legs straight up in the air. He kneels between her legs and raises her legs up so that her calves are resting on one of his shoulders. He leans forward and enters her.

what she can do: This is a great position for G-spot stimulation. She can pull her legs closer to her body to control the depth of penetration. Bringing her legs down and placing her feet on his chest will also let her control the tempo and depth of thrusts.

what he can do: He can place his hands on the bed or on either side of her body for support. This angle allows for deep penetration, so go slowly in the beginning to avoid discomfort and check in with her to make sure she is at ease.

> **BONUS!**
>
> It is a good idea to start slowly and gently when it comes to stimulating the G-spot, located on the front wall of the vagina. G-spot stimulation can even bring about female ejaculation in some women. Start slow, with light pressure via shallow thrusting, then move on to harder and deeper thrusting as she gets more aroused. Check in with her if her nonverbal cues and body language seem uncertain. Blended orgasms, from stimulating the clitoris and the G-spot at the same time, may be common for some women.

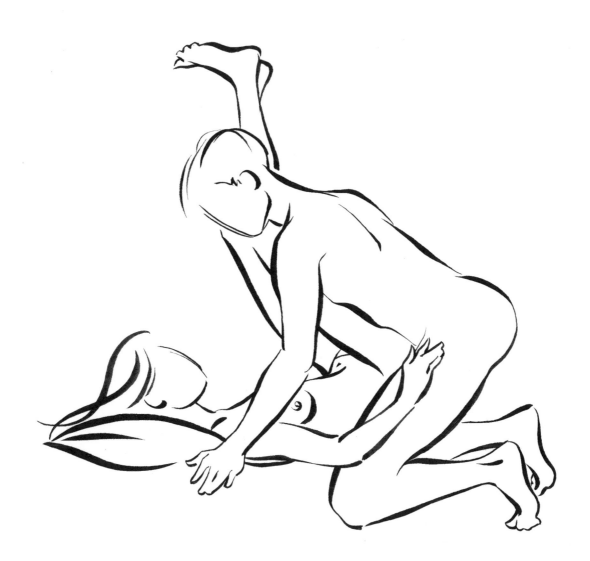

9.2 THE **BUTTER CHURNER**

This position may seem a bit excessive and is perhaps for couples looking to truly branch out of the norm. Lying on her back, she rolls her legs and torso up in the air so she is resting on her shoulders, with her arms down along the floor in front of her. He squats above her and penetrates her with quick and shallow thrusts. Deep and heavy thrusting is not recommended because her neck and shoulders are in a compromised position.

what she can do: She can place a pillow under her neck for comfort. For even better support, she can use a travel pillow, which wraps around the neck. If her core stomach muscles are stronger, this position will be easier. She may begin to feel lightheaded, as her legs are above her heart, so she needs to communicate with her partner when she is ready for something else.

what he can do: He should be prepared to go lightly and slowly. He should not attempt to sit on her bottom, but instead try to hold the majority of his weight in his thighs and legs. Essentially, he is in an elevated squat pose, above her. Both partners should have strength to maintain this position without putting undue stress on her neck.

> **BONUS!**
>
> With her legs above her heart, she may begin to feel lightheaded. Some people enjoy this sensation during sex and believe it leads to more intense orgasms.

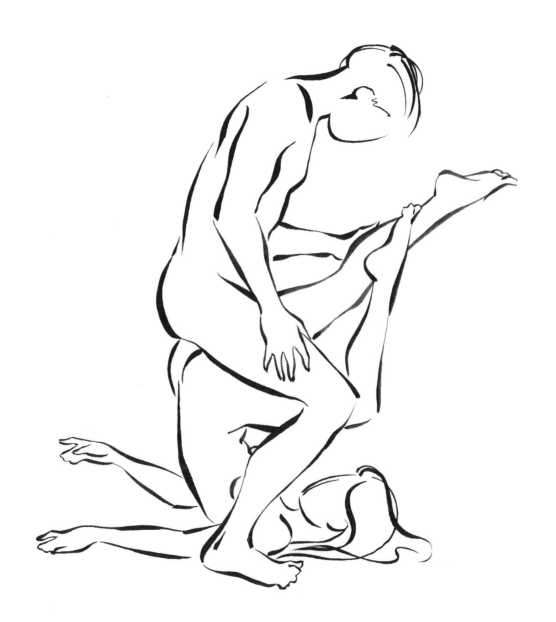

9.3 THE REVERSE **BUTTER CHURNER**

This position is slightly better than the Butter Churner for deep thrusting. Similar to the Butter Churner, she gets into a shoulder stand with her arms stretched out in front of her (yoga fans will better know this pose as the plow). In this variation, however, he is facing in the other direction, toward her front. This position may be a little easier for thrusting because it doesn't push directly on her neck. However, this is not a position to stay in for long periods of time, even with safety precautions.

what she can do: She can keep her legs together with her knees straight or bend her knees. If she is flexible, she can pull her knees down to the floor. This will give him greater access and give her an amazing stretch.

what he can do: He is on top in this pose and thus has a nice view. He also has full control, can watch his penis going in and out of her, and thus will likely be able to enjoy going slow and building up some tension in this pose. She is still folded up underneath him, and while deeper thrusting is possible, it still needs to be done with care.

> **BONUS!**
>
> As with all shoulder stand positions, if she has practice doing this pose, such as in yoga, or if she has strong core and back muscles, then these positions will be a lot easier, more enjoyable, and safer. She can practice shoulder stands and plow pose on her own, or even for a few minutes before sex. She may never look at yoga poses the same way again!

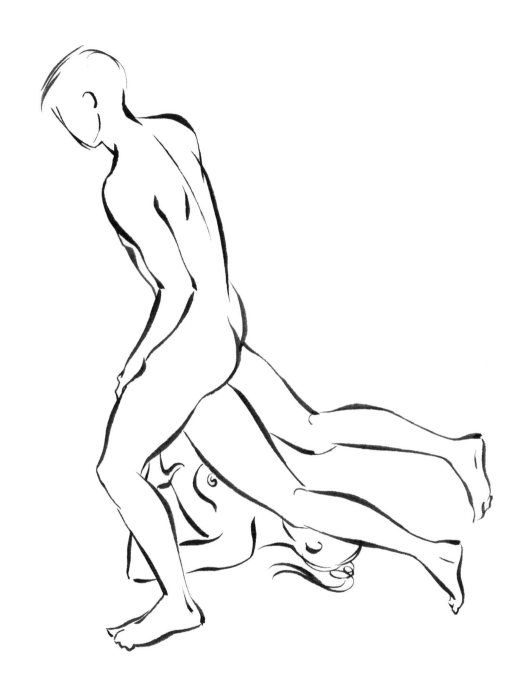

9.4 THE **DECK CHAIR**

This is a much easier and more relaxed variation of Shoulder Stand, and the focus is back on deep penetration. He sits and supports himself by leaning back on his hands with his legs outstretched in front of him. She lies back on a pillow facing him and props her feet up on his shoulders while arching her back. He can then enter her from this position.

what she can do: She can move the pillow under her bottom for slightly deeper penetration. She also has control of the depth and speed of penetration and can move her hips up and down, at the pace that suits her best. Her hands are free in this position, so she can reach down and stimulate her clitoris or the base of his penis. The arch in her back can help give her some control of her pubococcygeus (PC) muscles.

what he can do: Men often like this position because he has an excellent view of her vulva and his penis moving in and out of her vagina. He can also lean back and grab her thighs for really deep and hard penetration.

> **BONUS!**
>
> If he leans against a wall he will free up his hands for some clitoral stimulation, as he has easy access to her vulva. There are a lot of sex toys on the market that target the clitoris, such as the rabbit and bullet vibrators. Some light tickling with a feather is another option.

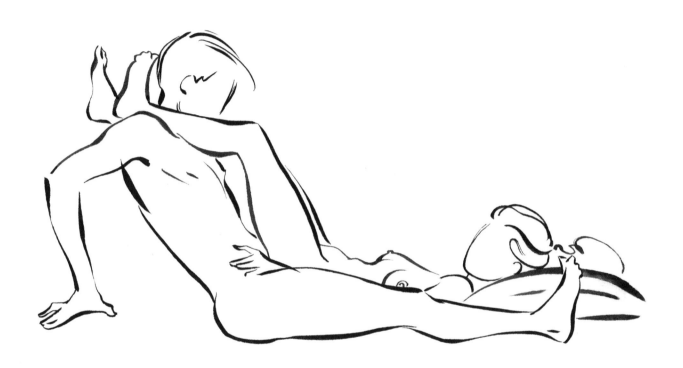

9.5 THE ROCK 'N ROLL

The Rock 'n Roll provides a slightly deeper folded variation than the Deck Chair. She lies on her back and swivels her hips up as if she is about to do a backwards roll, but not quite. He kneels in front of her and she rests her legs on his shoulders, while he supports some of his weight on the back of her legs. He can then enter her from this position. There is lot of intimacy in this variation. The couple's mouths and faces are close together, so kissing is easy, as is eye contact.

what she can do: The name suggests that there is some movement in this pose, and indeed her position makes it easy to rock back and forth.

what he can do: He can use his hands under her on each side to maintain a rocking motion, and the rocking aids penetration, bringing her body alternately closer to him and then farther away. He can position his knees underneath her to tilt and elevate her pelvis upward.

> **BONUS!**
>
> The upward tilt of her pelvis makes this a good position if trying to get pregnant. Semen pools at the base of her cervix, keeping the sperm in close proximity to her uterus and thus making fertilization more likely.

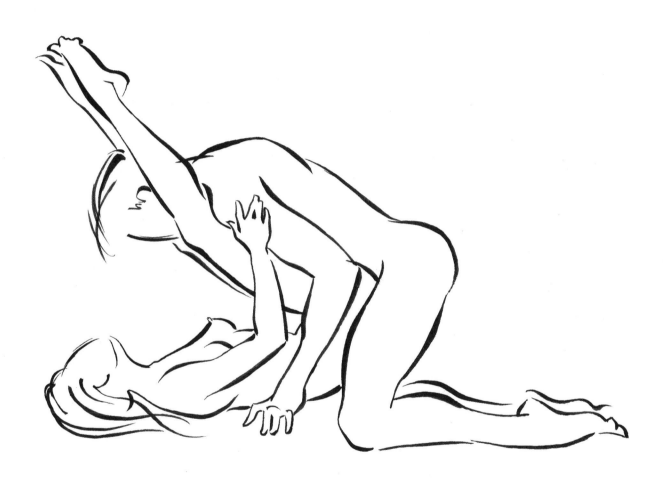

THE **SLIP**

In this angled Shoulder-Stand variation, his body is used as support, which gives him control and lets her sit back and enjoy the ride. She lies back with her torso completely flat and her head on a pillow. He kneels in front of her, and she tilts her hips and pelvis up and rests the back of her legs on his thighs. Her knees are bent and placed on each side of his hips, and her feet, if they reach, are on the bed. He enters her and then leans back with his arms behind him supporting his weight. The angle provides deep penetration with little effort.

what she can do: She has her hands free and can rest them on his hips to hold on or use them to stimulate herself. She can lift and position her entire body upward, grabbing on to his thighs or hips for support, as though she is about to do a backbend or the yoga position known as *bridge*. This brings her up higher and into a more direct angle with his penis. This also gives her some control, allows him some relief from doing all the work, and builds her thigh and stomach muscles. He gets a nice workout, too.

what he can do: For the most part, he controls the movement. He has a great view of the action and can also watch her face as she responds to his efforts.

BONUS!

Like many of the Shoulder Stand positions, this one works best if the couple is in relatively good shape. This brings a whole new level of motivation to maintaining an exercise routine that includes cardio and weight training. Even better, the couple can work out together, knowing what they are really training for!

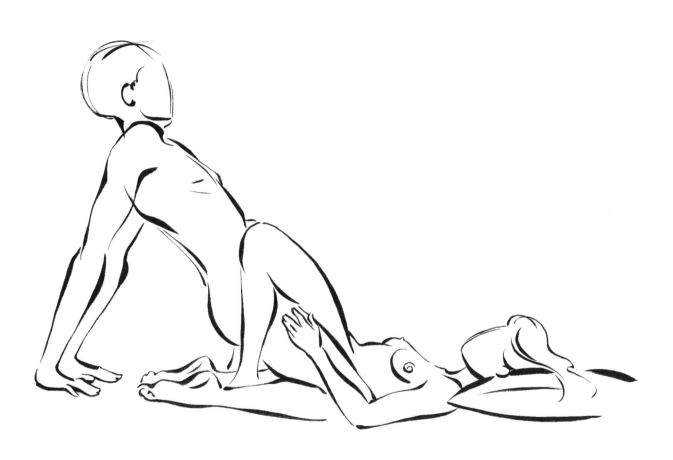

(9.7) THE G-FORCE

In this variation she is in a shoulder stand, but she is able to rest her hips on his body, which should make this position slightly less challenging for her. She lies on her back with her head and neck on a pillow and pulls her knees close to her chest. He kneels in front of her, and when she lifts up her hips and legs he catches her feet and holds them for the duration of this variation. Thrusting his hips forward, he can penetrate her while controlling the movement and supporting her balance.

what she can do: She can rest her feet on his chest while he grabs her hips. This will give him a little more control for some deeper and harder thrusting.

what he can do: He might like to have a pillow or blanket under his knees to provide some cushioning. Because he is holding her feet, he can move her legs together and apart and adjust their angle to hit all her erogenous zones.

> **BONUS!**
>
> She is at his mercy in this position. This can be a nice time for her to surrender to him and relinquish control over lovemaking. He can feel dominant in this position. Using role-play, dirty talk, and other elements of dominance and submission, they can take this to the next level. Perhaps he is a stern yoga instructor and she just can't get her shoulder stand aligned properly!

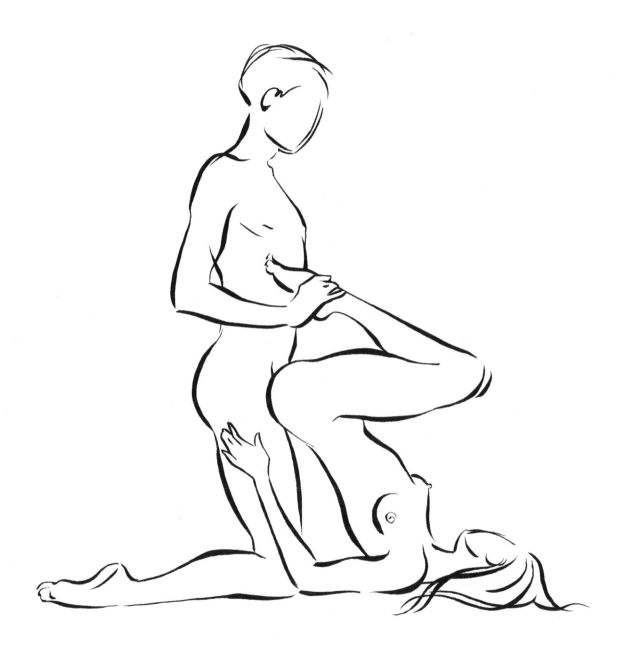

9.8 THE MAN ON **ALL FOURS**

In this variation, he is on his hands and knees, while she is in a modified shoulder stand or bridge pose. She lies on her back with her knees bent. He hovers above her on all fours. She lifts her hips up toward him, tilts her pelvis so it aligns with his, and then wraps her legs around his waist and lower back. Her arms are flat against the ground.

what she can do: She gets all her support from her upper arms and back in this position. If she has good upper body strength, this position will be much easier for her. She can push herself up and then release to let herself down a little, to create the depth of penetration that feels best for her.

what he can do: He can let her do most of the work. Being on all fours does not leave him much control, except maybe the movement in his pelvis. He can also sway back and forth to get a better angle.

> **BONUS!**
>
> In this position, she is in control of the thrusting and rhythm. If she wraps her arms around him, she relinquishes control and he will be in charge of the motion. The couple can take turns playing with the power imbalance, moving back and forth between dominance and submission.

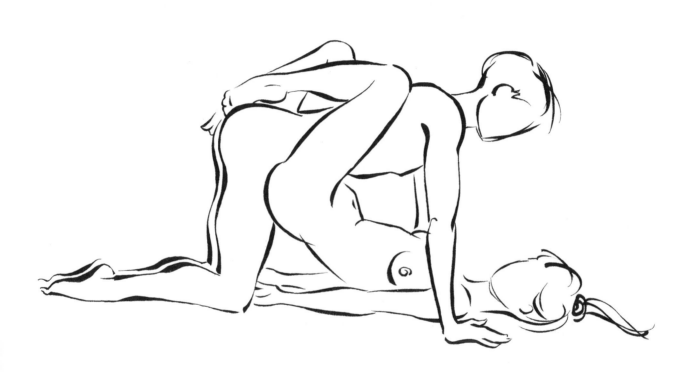

9.9 THE **SNAIL**

Another variation of the shoulder stand where he is on his knees is known as the Snail. From the Man on All Fours variation, he raises his upper body so that he is no longer in a flat back position; his torso is angled and his arms are beside her hips. She rolls up so that her bottom is in line with his pelvis. She throws her feet over his shoulders and uses his arms as support. He can then enter her from this position.

what she can do: This position should hit her G-spot and she can bring her knees closer to or farther away from her chest to vary the depth and angle of penetration.

what he can do: Depending on his arm strength, this variation may be hard to maintain. He can use quick, short, and shallow thrusts at first and then go in for deeper, longer thrusts, using his hips and core muscle strength to get the most out of deep penetration.

BONUS!

If both partners are comfortable, this is a great position for prolonged intercourse. To delay ejaculation, he can try this trick: Instead of going in and out, he can stay inside of her without thrusting for a few minutes. Then he swivels his hips, which has the effect of massaging her vagina while stimulating her clitoris, hands free, with his pelvic bone.

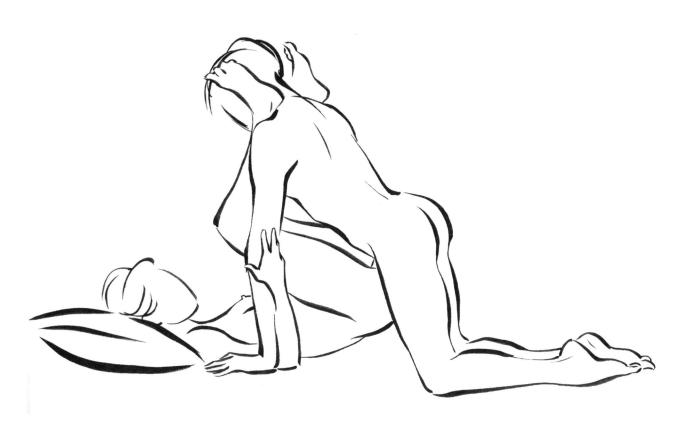

(9.10) THE **DOLPHIN**

This is reminiscent of the bridge pose in yoga and is excellent for G-spot stimulation. She lies on her back and spreads her legs. He kneels between them as she pushes her pelvis up toward him. Her head, neck, and shoulders remain resting on the bed while she arches her back. He helps support her by pulling her up by her hips and buttocks. He can then enter her from this position.

what she can do: If her stomach and upper arm muscles are strong, she will not need to use him for support as much. In this case, it is better for her to control the motion of thrusting.

what he can do: Gentle thrusts are key to the Dolphin variation. He should be careful not to go too hard or too fast. It is fine to go deep, as long as it is slow and steady. Hard, vigorous thrusts could be very dangerous in this position because of the strain it could put on her neck and shoulders.

> **BONUS!**
>
> Many of the more adventurous sex positions, such as the Dolphin, are reminiscent of yoga poses. This makes sense, as the Kama Sutra and yoga both arose in India. Never been one for yoga? Learning how to achieve and maintain a variety of poses that are also great sex positions just might change your mind.

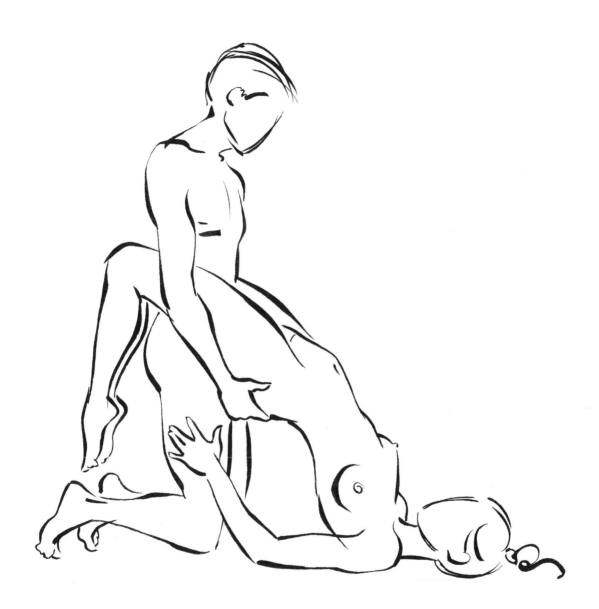

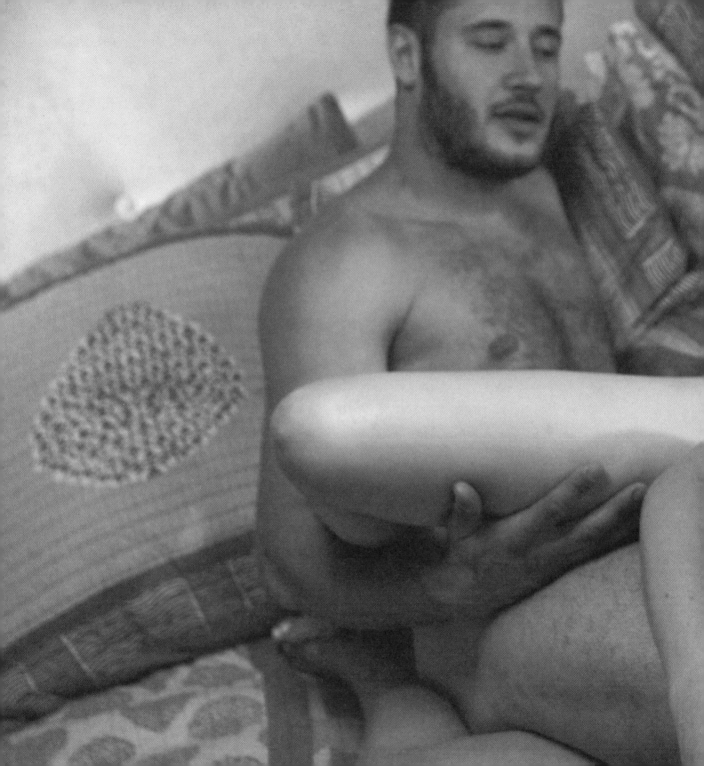

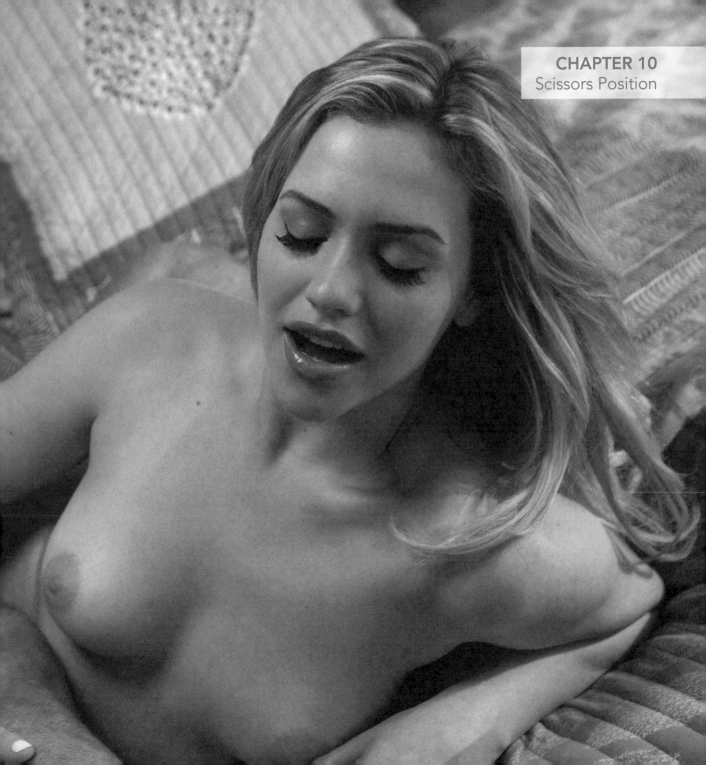

10

SCISSORS POSITION

IT WOULD SEEM THAT THE SCISSORS POSITION developed as the love child of the Doggy-Style and the Spooning sex positions. To get a better angle, the man places one of his legs in between both of her legs, thereby separating their two sets of legs and creating the well-known Scissors position. All the twists and turns of this classic position can create an exciting and much-needed diversion for couples trying to spruce up their sex life.

Scissoring is one position that is stimulating when clothes are on. The rocking motion of scissoring combined with the friction from the clothes can be extremely erotic. It's great for a couple just starting out. But long-term couples who engage in "dry humping," or sex that does not necessarily lead to or end in intercourse, orgasm, or ejaculation, will find that it encourages them to focus on the sensuous aspects of sexuality and break out of the monotony of needing to have penetration every time they become intimate with one another. This can open the door for a lot more fun and varied exploration.

The Scissors looks more difficult to get into than it actually is, but it does require some maneuvering until the couple finds a comfortable position. Using pillows under her back or hips can help make the position a little more comfortable for her.

How to Do It

She lies on her side with one leg stacked on top of the other. He lies on his side facing her back or her bottom with his head close to her feet. She raises her top leg and bends it so that he will be able to slip his top leg in between to directly access her vagina. Then he puts his lower leg under her lower leg and moves toward her. Her lower leg is between his legs. From here he can enter her and start thrusting.

benefits for her

If his leg or pelvis rubs her in the right way, it will massage her clitoris. The angle, depending on his size, shape, and depth of thrusting, can also stimulate her G-spot.

As with every sex pose, being relaxed and comfortable is the key. Since he is in charge it can help to ride along with his movement. But if she wants to have a little more control, she can use her body to thrust back and forth with him. She can grab on to his top leg to get some leverage and to thrust back onto him. She can also touch her clitoris or stimulate her breasts and nipples.

benefits for him

Pulling her top leg toward his chest will give him more leverage for thrusting. Try this position with the bed against the wall. He can put his hand against the wall, which will act as support. Also, try this position on a couch or sofa, so he can put one leg on the floor, which will also give him a leg-up on support.

A BIT OF HISTORY

Commonly referred to as tribadism, tribbing, or frottage, scissoring originates from the act of rubbing one's genitals against another's body or genitals without penetration or exchange of body fluids. Scissoring can be done with clothes on, providing friction and stimulation of the clitoris. Men may also rub the tip of their penis against various parts of their partner's body to stimulate and arouse them both. In ancient Greece, the word *tiribo* meant "to rub" and *tribas* was used to describe "a woman who practices unnatural vice with herself or with other women." Today, scissoring is commonly associated with lesbian sex, thanks to the popular animated series *South Park*, but lesbians are not the only ones to scissor. Scissoring can mimic Missionary, Woman-on-Top, and Doggy-Style positions, with clothes on or off, and with or without penetration.

10.1 THE CATHERINE WHEEL

In this variation, the man and woman sit facing each other, and then the woman reaches and wraps her legs around his body. For support, she leans back on her hands and pushes herself slightly up off the ground/bed. The man leans back and supports himself on one elbow and wraps the opposite leg around her body. This leg has the effect of support for him to hold her in place and use it for leverage to initiate penetration, but his arm that he is leaning on is really doing much of the work. This might not be the most comfortable position if the couple is aiming for deep, fast thrusting. It lends itself to slow, long penetration with some eye gazing. Both can use pillows under their bottoms if it feels better.

what she can do: She may be able to reach over and stimulate her clitoris, or her clitoris may naturally rub against his body.

what he can do: The angle is great for hitting her G-spot, because the shallow areas of her vagina will get the most stimulation. He can lean forward or backward to get just the right angle.

> **BONUS!**
>
> This is a great position for her to pleasure herself and give him a show, and he is in the perfect position to watch every move. Mutual masturbation is always a sexy and erotic addition to any couple's repertoire, and it shows each other what you like. If this position gets too uncomfortable, he can take his penis out and both can continue touching themselves for each other's visual pleasure.

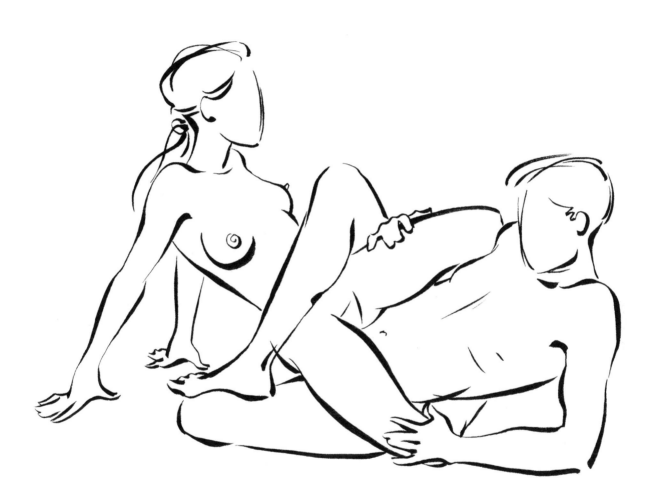

10.2 SIDEWAYS **SCISSORS**

There are two ways to pull off the Sideways Scissors. In the first one, she lies on her side facing him, with her head propped up on one elbow. He lies perpendicular to her and places both of his legs between her legs. Her bottom leg is under his thigh. In the second one, he faces her on his knees, taking her bottom leg beneath his butt so he can move forward and enter her. Both versions provide an interesting angle for penetration.

what she can do: She can adjust her angle, sit forward or backward, or prop herself up on some pillows to achieve the right angle. She can also thrust her vulva against his leg to stimulate her clitoris.

what he can do: With her leg underneath him, she may get uncomfortable or feel like her leg is getting crushed by his body weight. He can leverage himself up on his legs, using his thigh muscles, to alleviate some of the discomfort. Placing a pillow between them might also work.

> **BONUS!**
>
> If this position gets too tiring or doesn't seem to be working, she is in the perfect position to give him a hand job. He can simply pull out and let her talented hands go to work.

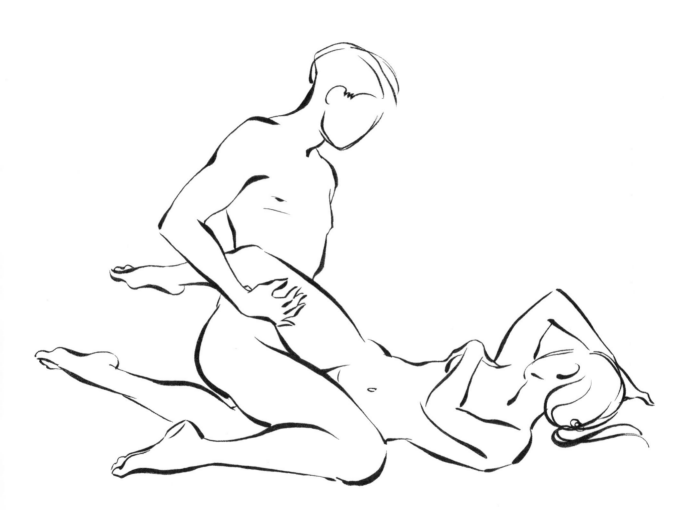

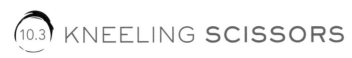

10.3 KNEELING **SCISSORS**

In this variation, there is a bit more comfort and her G-spot may see a lot more action. She lies face down with one side slightly raised, her legs straight out behind her. She can rest her head on an arm or pillow if it feels more comfortable. He kneels right behind her bottom, with one of his legs between her legs, where he can penetrate her.

what she can do: Her vagina is not as easily accessible in this pose, but that might make this feel like a tighter fit. She can slide her top leg up higher so that it is bent. This will make it easier for him to enter her and also give him a good view of the action. Raising her knee also adjusts the angle to target the G-spot. She can also slide her front hand down and stimulate her clitoris.

what he can do: With his hand he can lift her body up to one side, if this makes it easier for penetration. He can slide his outer knee up higher along her body to get a better angle. His hands are free as well, so he can use his fingers or a vibrator to give her more intense stimulation in this position. He can also give her some light spanks on the bottom to build intensity.

> **BONUS!**
>
> This is a great position for anal play. While penetrating her vagina, he can insert his finger into her anus. This does not need to go very deep at all. Keep it shallow. The combination of having her G-spot, clitoris, and anus stimulated at the same time can take her over the edge.

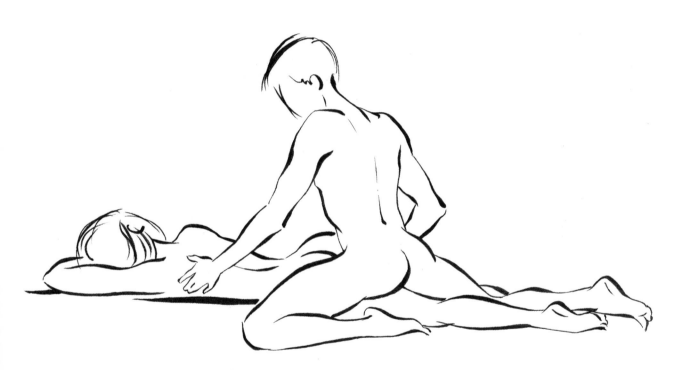

10.4 SCORPION **SCISSORS**

This sex position is not one for the faint of heart. But, for those looking for adventure and novelty, it is a must-try. The woman lies on her back, with her legs apart, and the man penetrates her while facing in the opposite direction. She then puts her legs on his back, and he can support himself on his forearms.

what she can do: She can grab a hold of his knees to aid in the thrusting. She is also in a great position to stimulate his testicles very gently, maybe by lightly rubbing her clitoris against them. It is important to remember that testicles are extremely sensitive, so a light touch is all he needs. The element of surprise can be exciting for him, too.

what he can do: Deep, fast thrusting is not the mainstay of this pose. But this is a good thing because it gives him the opportunity to do something different. He can try making circles or figure eights with his hips. He can also try simply holding his penis inside her for longer periods of time.

BONUS!

Penetration without the thrusting motion, or with the goal of ejaculation, is a practice commonly associated with Tantra and was also used by sex researchers Masters and Johnson to get couples to focus on sensation and not orgasm. Sex therapists use this technique to help men gain control of the erections and ejaculations, to extend sex play, and to encourage the couple to enjoy pleasure without an end goal. When the man and woman practice this without the goal of orgasm, they focus on the heat their bodies are exchanging, which in turn increases tension and arousal. While this may seem counterintuitive, this can ultimately lead both partners to even more explosive orgasms.

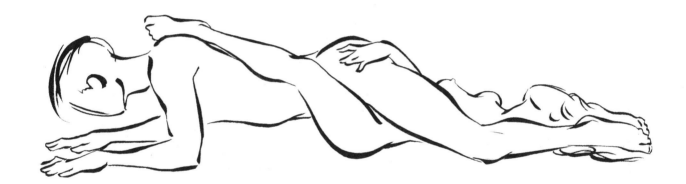

10.5 BOTH LEGS UP **SCISSORS**

In this position, the woman lies on her back, ideally on a table or countertop. The man faces her, standing at the edge of the table. The woman places her legs on his shoulders, and he holds on to her ankles. He spreads her legs apart and enters her. Then he crosses and uncrosses her legs in front of him as he thrusts. Though not an easy position, the opening and closing of her legs causes shifts in her pelvic muscles, which will give him the sensation of tightness alternating with openness. This position also allows for deep penetration.

what she can do: Even though he is doing most of the work, having some strength in her legs will help this position along. Also, because her hands are free she can stimulate her breasts, nipples, and clitoris, which will not only feel good to her but also be a pleasure for him to watch.

what he can do: He gets a great view of her whole body, and he can communicate where he wants her to touch next.

> **BONUS!**
>
> This is a great position to take out of the bedroom and have a little fun with. She can sit on the hood of a car (parked in the garage with the garage door down, of course!) and he, perhaps a horny auto mechanic, can "service" her after he looks under her hood.

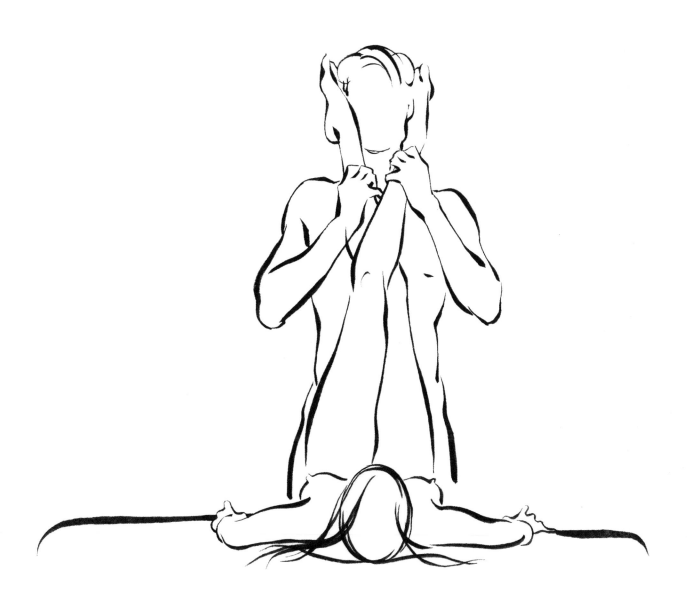

(10.6) THE X POSITION

In this exciting and only slightly challenging variation of Scissors, the couple sits on the bed facing each other with their legs outstretched. She lifts one of her legs over his and he lifts his other leg over hers. Then the two scoot close together so he can put his penis inside her. She can lie back while he sits up, and then they can alternate him lying down while she sits up. They can hold, massage, and caress each other's feet as well.

what she can do: Penetration will likely be shallow in this position, which can stimulate her G-spot. She can adjust the height of her body to get the right angle. She can also put a leg over one of his shoulders.

what he can do: He can scoot forward and back on his butt to increase arousal and aid in the thrusting. He can also lift his hips slightly while resting on his hands if that gives him more leverage.

BONUS!

Hold hands. This may give the couple more leverage while also bringing tenderness to the position. They can take turns like a seesaw, one sitting up and the other lying back, as they pull each other by the hands to keep the rhythm going. If they find a nice pace the result could be prolonged stimulation of her G-spot and the tip of his penis.

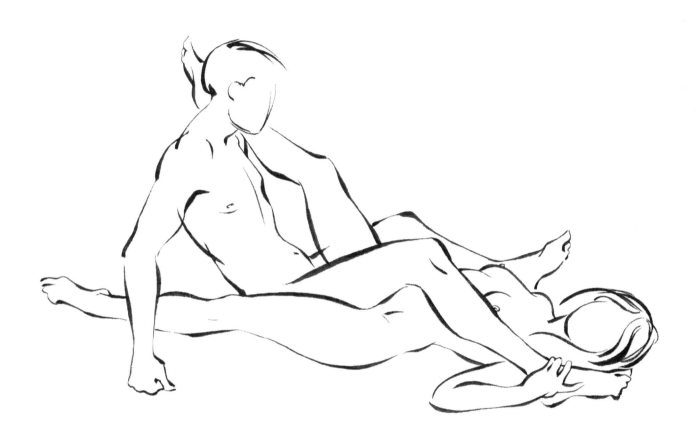

ROCKING **SCISSORS**

This is a nice transition position, or a more relaxing position because it forces the couple to slow down. From Sideways Scissors, he straightens his legs so he can put his face close to hers, and then he holds her and together they roll to the side. If he is flexible, he might be able to do this with his knees bent, but straight legs might be more comfortable. The couple can also roll while he still has his penis in her. Their legs are intertwined and their chests pressed against each other. She has one leg in between his, and her other leg is on the outside of his body.

what they can do: Go slow. This is an opportunity to wind down and reconnect. Make eye contact, kiss each other's necks, have a make-out session. Rock back and forth, which will stimulate her G-spot and clitoris simultaneously because his pelvis is rubbing against hers.

> **BONUS!**
>
> This is an excellent position for taking a break when things get too intense and either partner wants to delay orgasm. Before the point of no return, he can take his penis out and continue to stimulate her clitoris before resuming intercourse. This will slow things down and prolong the excitement.

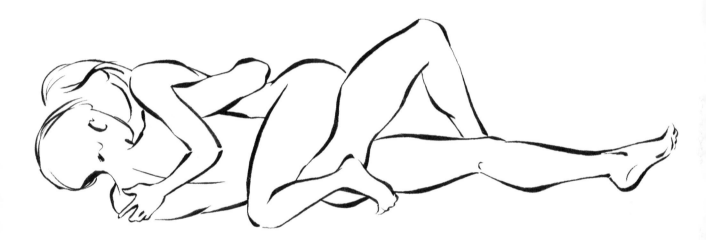

(10.8) THE **SPIDER**

The Spider is another not-so-easy Scissor-esque position that may seem like a game of Twister. Both are seated on the bed with their legs toward the other. They use their arms behind them to support themselves. They then crawl or scoot toward each other, like spiders. Her hips are between his legs, and her knees are bent. Her feet are outside of his hips and flat on the bed. He can then enter her from this position. During intercourse, the couple can rock back and forth.

what she can do: If she can balance she can use one hand to guide his penis inside of her. She can push her hips toward his pelvis to allow him better access for penetration.

what he can do: He can watch her body maneuvering into this position. He gets a great view of her vulva and his penis going in and out of her. He can also make eye contact with her to increase the intimacy and connection. Since he has more support he can control the thrusting as well.

> **BONUS!**
>
> Try this one with clothes on. Or if penetration is tricky, he can rub his penis against her clitoris. Building heat and friction is fun in this position.

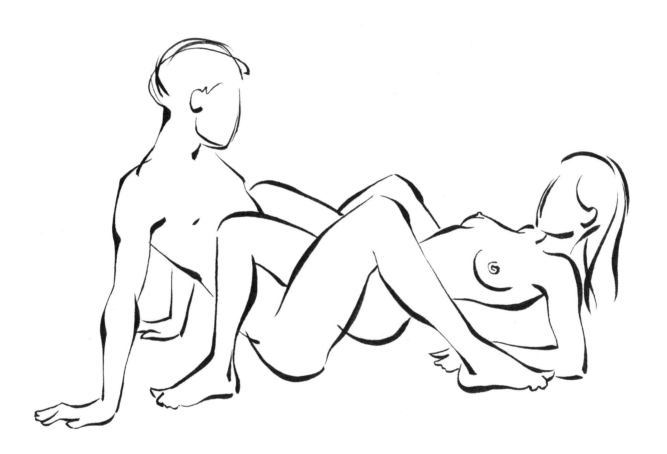

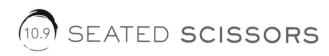

10.9 SEATED **SCISSORS**

The man sits down on a chair to get started, with his legs stretched out in front of him. She climbs onto his lap and assumes a similar position, stretching her legs out straight in front of her, and thus behind him. He holds on to her arms and she holds on to his for support. She can begin by leaning back to gain some control and to insert his penis in her vagina.

what she can do: She can guide the position as fast or as slow as she wants by moving her body back and forth on top of him. Their legs look like a pair of scissors on each side. Her core strength is what drives this position.

what he can do: He holds her in place by holding down her arms. Because she is in control, he can just sit back and enjoy the ride.

> **BONUS!**
>
> This is a great time for her to bring out her inner dominatrix. If they are in an office or in a chair similar to an office chair, she might play the demanding boss and he is her hapless assistant who just accidentally deleted all her files and lost that major client's contract. He might get fired unless he can find a way to please her, and fast . . .

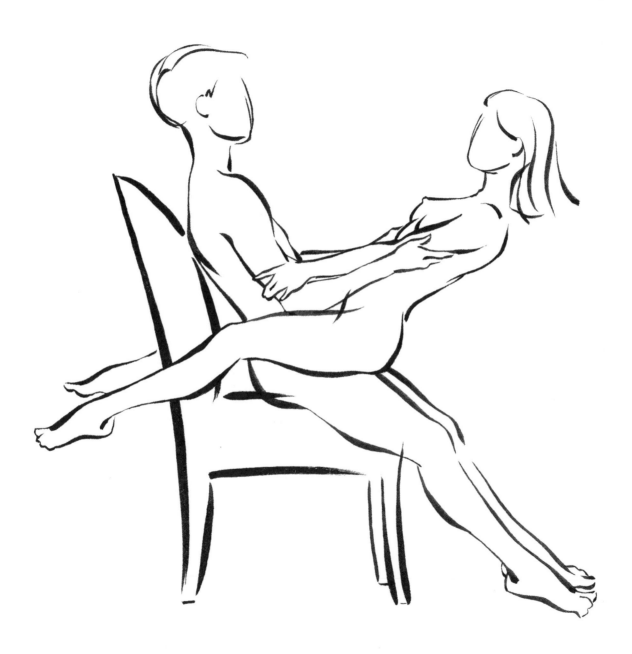

(10.10) STANDING **SCISSORS**

This position is perfect for an impromptu get-together. For some quick action, the couple can just remove their pants and keep their top half clothed. Standing face to face, with their legs interlaced—one of her legs is in between his and her other leg is outside his thigh—he penetrates her. Or they can keep their clothes on and enjoy some dry humping.

what she can do: If there is too much of a height difference, she can put on some high heels to make this position easier. Standing on something or doing this on the stairs might work, too. She can also wear a skirt with no panties to tantalize him with her readiness for sex.

what he can do: He can spread his legs out to bring his height down a bit, back her up against a wall, or grab her ass and rub her clitoris against his leg.

> **BONUS!**
>
> This is a great position for a dimly lit dance-floor seduction, as it allows for a lot of eye gazing and deep kissing, with their bodies pressed close together. They'll have their clothes on, but that's okay—they can just press their crotches together as they sway to the music.

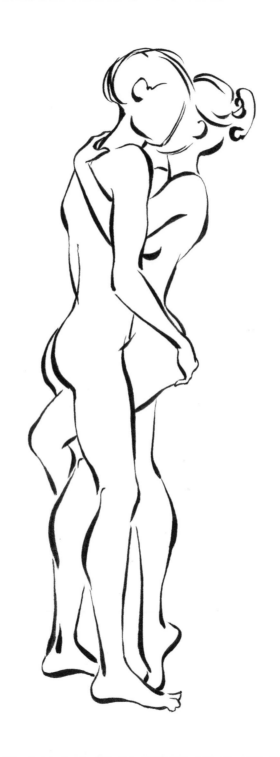

CONCLUSION

I hope that you found something helpful in these pages to add to your sexual repertoire. This book is a reference guide meant to inspire exploration. As you go back
and revisit the positions, you will learn something new or be reminded of something
you want to try again. Although the positions may seem simple enough, there are
some gems that are only enjoyed with more in-depth experience—or strength, flexibility, and trust. This book is not intended to be used like a checklist. Instead, treat
your sexuality as a lifelong journey—and enjoy the ride!!

ABOUT THE AUTHOR

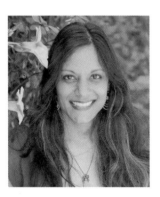

MOUSHUMI GHOSE is a licensed marriage and
family therapist. An activist and an advocate for
sexual freedom for many years, Mou is a member
of AASECT (American Association of Sex Educators,
Counselors and Therapists) and KAP (Kink Aware
Professionals). She writes for YourTango, Good-
Therapy, and has been quoted in *American Curves
Magazine*, *Men's Fitness*, *Men's Health*, eHarmony,
Hustler Hollywood, PsychCentral, and more. Visit
her online at www.lasextherapist.com.

ACKNOWLEDGMENTS

This book was made possible with the support, encouragement, and help of some
very amazing and integral people.

First of all, I want to recognize my clients. Watching my clients learn, grow, and
change provides me with the insight to do the work that I do. Without them none of
this is needed or possible.

I want to thank Fair Winds Press for giving me this opportunity to share my knowledge, and for providing a much-needed avenue for sex-positive education. I'd like

to thank the team for making the editing and publishing process smooth, fun, and something to look forward to. Specifically, I want to thank Jill Alexander for taking a chance on me, as well as supporting and guiding me throughout the process. Marissa Giambrone for her patience, vision, and flexibility during the illustration process, John Gettings for his support in finalizing the book, Karen Levy, and Amy Paradysz for their insight and clarity during the editing process.

For helping me map out all the positions with sticky notes, for attempting to mimic positions with me, helping me with mundane questions in the middle of the night, not to mention tedious editing, grammar, proofreading; and for tolerating and supporting me when I would get stressed out, I want to thank my partner Jarrod Kenney.

A humongous thanks to my parents for gently guiding me and providing me with the avenue for higher education, for allowing me to be me, make my own choices and mistakes, for believing in me, supporting me, and not asking a lot of questions about my profession!

I want to thank Amie Harwick for her generosity, recognition, ongoing support, courageous spirit, and for introducing me to Quiver.

I would love to acknowledge the sex-positive community in Los Angeles. There is a growing group of amazing, insightful, and intelligent sexual health proponents whose knowledge and support are not only inspiring but also encouraging and great reminders that this work we do is needed.

There are a few amazing sex-positive people, whom I consider to be my peers, whom I look to for support, who inspire my work on a very regular basis, and encourage me to embrace my values, open my mind, and get me to think about sex and relationships in brand new ways: Jenoa Harlow, Laurie Bennett-Cook, Damon Holzum, and Shai Rotem.

Thank you to Heather Cozen, for her patience in working with me as a newbie clinical supervisor, then for sticking with me for five years, and especially for her thoughtful, caring, and wise sex-positive spirit.

I also would like to acknowledge the mental health community at Pepperdine University for recognizing and welcoming my visions in the field of sexuality and allowing me the space to educate and expand within this field, nurturing both education and growth—and specifically Dr. Norma Scarborough at Alliant University for providing me with ample teaching and educating opportunities.

And finally, thanks to my band of rebels, Moshe Ben-Yosef and Jenae Heitkamp, for supporting me and being believers of change.

INDEX